Empathy Has no Rank

By

Dr. Raheem Lay

EMPATHY HAS NO RANK

Copyright © 2023 Dr. Raheem Lay

All rights reserved.

ISBN: 9798394496448

DEDICATION

This book pays tribute to the many events that have helped me evolve into the military officer and leader I am today, with each one serving as a milestone on my path to personal development. I pay homage to Erika Lay, my devoted wife, whose courage and insight continue to motivate me. To my daughters, Nyree and Nevaeh Lay, you are the embodiment of all that is good in my world and the driving force behind my desire to be a better leader and human being. May the lessons encapsulated in these pages serve me and all of us as we navigate the complexities of leadership and life.

EMPATHY HAS NO RANK

CONTENTS

	Acknowledgments	i
	Introduction	7
1	Empathy 101	10
2	Empathetic Leadership	17
3	The Military Paradigm	21
4	Shifting Perspectives	39
5	From Boots to Heart	45
6	Barracks to Battlefield	55
7	The Empathy Ripple Effect	59
8	Beyond Rank	63
9	Empathy in Crisis	67
10	Empathy Void	72
11	Empathy Skills for Leaders	84
	Conclusion	103

EMPATHY HAS NO RANK

ACKNOWLEDGMENTS

I want to express my heartfelt thanks to the US Air Force and the outstanding individuals who work with me. The institution has served as my military career's canvas and the forging ground for my leadership, service, and empathy knowledge.

A special thank you goes to those who have stood beside me during the emotionally challenging times and setbacks that are an inevitable part of a life of service. Your unwavering support, wisdom, and encouragement have been my bedrock, helping me transform obstacles into growth opportunities.

I am also incredibly appreciative of the mentors and classmates whose compassionate leadership in a time of difficulty has served as an example to follow and aspirations. Your capacity to maintain compassion despite the most challenging facts has irrevocably influenced how I lead.

Finally, this book belongs to the leadership who model empathy in everything they do. It is an ongoing reminder that a team's strength rests in its solidarity, developed by compassion and understanding. This book is for you.

INTRODUCTION

Leadership entails more than just issuing instructions, managing resources, and ensuring compliance. Effective leadership is fundamentally about understanding people, interacting with them, and creating an atmosphere where they may thrive. The need for empathy in leadership cannot be stressed in the context of the United States military, where the stakes can be exceedingly high. Regardless of rank or position, empathetic leaders are more suited to create teamwork, boost morale, and improve overall unit effectiveness. Empathy empowers a leader to understand another person's perspective, put oneself in their shoes, and behave in a considerate and wise way.

Before understanding why empathy is vital for good leadership, it is important to emphasize what can go wrong when it is lacking. For this debate, take Colonel Smith, the highest-ranking officer in his Battalion. Colonel Smith was well-decorated and had a wealth of experience in tactical operations. He was incredibly skilled, diligent, and technically outstanding in his profession. He was, however, also infamous for his sarcastic demeanor and lack of emotional intelligence.

Under his command, service members felt devalued and unheard regularly. Such issues as granting short leaves for family emergencies or adjusting mealtimes to meet the group's requirements were a growing source of resentment among his subordinates. Colonel Smith regarded these issues as distractions from the mission and refused to address them, widening the chasm between himself and those he led. He believed that the role of a commander was to command, and the part of a soldier was to follow.

Colonel Smith's leadership style lacked empathy,

negatively impacting the unit's performance. Fearing dismissal or derision, service members were less likely to share insightful ideas or feedback. This lack of open communication affected the operational fitness of the unit negatively. Perhaps even more alarming was its effect on morale. service members became disengaged not only from their duties but also from the unit's overall mission. When a high-stakes operation presented itself, the dearth of cohesion and trust became apparent. The unit's poor performance led to preventable errors and mission failure.

The Colonel Smith example demonstrates the detrimental effects that can result from a lack of empathy in a leader, which is particularly troublesome in a demanding and unpredictable environment like the military. When those in leadership roles fail to understand or consider the points and opinions of the individuals they have been tasked with leading, the consequences can be highly detrimental. Leadership that lacks empathy can damage employees' morale, decrease productivity, and even lead to mission failure.

It is not the role of empathy in the military to babysit service members or avoid making difficult decisions. It is about acknowledging the human factors that are frequently and deeply integrated into the functioning of efficient military organizations. Empathetic leaders can monitor the emotional state of everyone in the company, from the top ranks all the way down. They can recognize instances of diminished morale, periods of heightened stress, and circumstances where a small act of kindness could wield a profound influence.

Leaders must know their staff members' psychological and emotional health in a profession where actions frequently have life-or-death repercussions. In addition, it concerns preserving the military's fundamental tenets and the well-being of women and men who have sacrificed their lives in the line of service. No matter their position or status, all leaders must learn how to lead effectively through developing empathy. Empathy is not just a "soft skill" but a critical competency.

Military leaders at every echelon can potentially enhance their success, effectiveness, and compassion by dedicating the effort to grasp the significance of empathy. Through this commitment, they can achieve the objectives of their missions and uphold the broader moral and ethical obligations intertwined with the weighty mantle of leadership.

CHAPTER 1:

EMPATHY 101:

UNDERSTANDING THE BASICS

The initiation of any transformative endeavor frequently necessitates the undertaking of a crucial initial action. The initiation of my pursuit of compassionate military leadership did not occur within an academic setting but rather transpired during my leadership experiences. Before venturing into the theoretical underpinnings, it is essential to gain a comprehensive understanding of the essence of empathy. The term in question holds significance beyond its everyday usage in leadership discourse. Effective and empathetic leadership is the fundamental pillar of organizational success.

So, what exactly is empathy?

Empathy refers to the cognitive and affective ability to adopt another individual's perspective, comprehend their emotional state, and potentially experience a similar emotional response. Engaging with another individual's circumstances is more than simple intellectualization; it entails personal experiential involvement. I recall supervising a training session where newly enlisted individuals encountered difficulties while attempting a physically demanding assignment. Experiencing pity upon comprehending their predicament, my recollection of the initial days of my training, characterized by sweat and the struggle to suppress tears, engendered a sense of empathy.

The construct of empathy comprises three primary components: cognitive empathy, emotional empathy, and compassionate empathy.

1. Cognitive Empathy: This dimension of cognitive empathy focuses on perspective-taking. It refers to understanding another individual's thoughts and emotions without necessarily experiencing them oneself. Cognitive empathy is referred to as "walking a mile in their shoes."

Assume you are the flight leader, and Alex, one of your service members, has been routinely performing poorly during drills. You might have just told Alex off for not keeping up with the squad, but you chose to take a cognitive empathy approach. To understand the problem, you first talk one-on-one with the person. You learn through the conversation that Alex has been through a challenging divorce and struggles to juggle military obligations, court appearances, and child custody disputes.

Even though you have never gone through a divorce yourself, you attempt to comprehend the emotional and practical toll it is having on Alex. You consider the strain of working with lawyers, the emotional toll of a broken relationship, and the difficulty meeting professional expectations. Although you are not experiencing Alex's emotions, you understand how complicated their feelings and thoughts are.

This is an example of cognitive empathy. You have mentally traveled a mile in Alex's shoes, comprehending their problems without necessarily bearing their emotional load. And by adopting a different viewpoint, you can lead more skillfully. For example, you could temporarily alter Alex's training plan or provide him with tools to deal with stress. Even if you cannot help Alex with his personal issues, knowing their viewpoint can help you create a more encouraging and productive workplace.

2. Emotional Empathy: This is the affective aspect of empathy, where you share another person's emotions. If a teammate is ecstatic after performing well in an exercise, you feel similarly elated. If they are discouraged by a setback, you think again. This emotional synchronicity is what emotional empathy is about.

Consider yourself a member of a military team preparing

for a high-stakes mission. The atmosphere is apprehensive; everyone knows the current mission's significance. A member of your team is tasked with strategizing a crucial aspect of the operation. She has been under considerable stress and is visibly tense. She is noticeably relieved and pleased when her plan is unanimously approved after she presents it to the team.

Here is where emotional empathy enters the picture: You find yourself here as you observe Sarah's delighted expression. Her joy is infectious, elevating the spirits of the entire team. You did not plan the event or carry her burden, but you feel her happiness as if it were your own.

Advance to the date of the operation. Despite meticulous planning and high hopes, something needs to be fixed, and Sarah's part of the operation encounters a setback. You can't help but feel your stomach settling when you look into her eyes. Even though you weren't in charge of that specific area of the procedure, you find yourself sympathizing with her dissatisfaction. You stoop a little due to the chamber's weight pressing your shoulders.

This is an empathetic emotion. You are not merely aware of Sarah's emotions; you are experiencing them alongside her. This emotional synchronization is potent. Not only can it strengthen relationships, but it can also foster a cohesive team dynamic that enhances mutual support and comprehension. And in sectors like the military, where emotional stakes are often high, such a bond can substantially improve morale and effectiveness.

3. Compassionate Empathy: This exemplifies the manifestation of empathy. The demonstration of understanding and feeling for someone else's state stretches beyond the simple ability to grasp, as it constrains people to give helpful help when conditions warrant it.

Consider yourself as the commanding officer of a military unit deployed in a foreign country. One squad member, namely John, has recently been informed of the critical condition of his father residing in his hometown. It is observed that John's performance is adversely affected, as evidenced by his diminished focus and shorter response times relative to his typical performance. One can comprehend the individual's experience of worry and emotional distress by employing cognitive empathy. Through the expertise of a passionate heart, one actively shares in another individual's concerns and feelings of sorrow, cultivating a personal sense of weightiness and respect.

But compassionate empathy takes you a step further.

You are determined to act instead of merely understanding or sharing John's emotions. You sit down and talk with him, suggesting that he be temporarily relocated closer to home. You also navigate the bureaucracy to expedite his emergency leave request. On top of that, you rearrange the team's responsibilities to compensate for his absence without compromising the mission.

Your actions here are motivated by compassion. You no longer merely comprehend or sense John's emotional state; you feel compelled to take action to alleviate his anxiety. This action provides John with immediate respite and reinforces the vibrant fabric of your entire team. They observe that their leader understands and shares their emotions and takes decisive action when necessary. This fosters a community of trust and respect for one another, which is crucial for any team's performance, especially in high-stakes settings like the military.

Therefore, compassionate empathy involves more than just 'feeling' but also 'doing.' It is empathy that manifests itself in actions that seek to alleviate someone's emotional distress or solve their problem. Moreover, this type of empathy is frequently the most profound, leaving a lasting impression on those it affects.

You may question, "Why should a military leader like me care about empathy?" I can assure you that empathy is not limited to counselors and elementary school instructors. It is essential for anyone aspiring to lead effectively, whether in a military platoon, corporate boardroom, or even at a blackjack table.

In a military context, the concept of empathy pertains not to the notion of being a lenient or permissive leader, but rather to the comprehension of the complex interplay of human behavior, requirements, and sentiments within one's squad. The level of comprehension described can enhance confidence, enhance group unity, and provide essential perspectives for the process of making decisions. In essence, empathy emerges as a strategic resource that can strengthen one's leadership abilities and make a substantial contribution to the achievement of organizational objectives.

It is essential to avoid conflating empathy with a panacea. This technology does not confer invulnerability nor guarantee victory in conflicts. However, its potential lies in enhancing your leadership skills, resulting in compliance, authentic admiration, and allegiance from your team. The undisclosed formula can elevate one's leadership abilities from conventional to exceptional.

Adopting an empathetic leadership style is replete with various obstacles and difficulties. There may arise situations in which the emotional burden becomes overwhelming or prompts one to question the intrinsic value of engaging in sympathetic interactions. Remembering empathy doesn't denote vulnerability during challenging moments is essential. Instead, it showcases a person's resilience. While it grants a deeper comprehension of the inherent complexities of the human condition, this understanding doesn't imply a relinquishment of control. Ultimately, leadership, especially in the military's high-stakes and emotionally charged context, is not solely about developing resilience but about embodying genuine and courageous humanity.

CHAPTER 2

EMPATHETIC LEADERSHIP: WHY IT MATTERS

Empathy is commonly perceived as a comforting and soothing idea, offering temporary solace within a tumultuous context. Nevertheless, the significance of this concept goes beyond providing emotional comfort and carries substantial importance in the realm of leadership, namely in the context of military operations. Considering the prevailing perception of the military as an establishment characterized by principles such as discipline, resilience, and hierarchical power, it is reasonable to raise inquiries regarding the relevance and suitability of empathy in this particular context.

Leadership can be defined as the process of effectively motivating individuals towards the achievement of common goals. Attempting to achieve a goal without a comprehensive awareness of the elements that drive one's team, the concerns that bring them distress, or the desires that urge them is worth considering. Engaging in such a pursuit would resemble traversing nautical regions devoid of the assistance provided by a navigational instrument known as a compass.

Empathy is crucial in guiding leaders to navigate skillfully across the complex landscape of human emotions and cognitive processes. This approach facilitates a more profound comprehension of team members, surpassing the constraints imposed by hierarchical positions, to acknowledge each soldier as a distinct combination of ambitions, concerns, and capacities. By recognizing this intricate aspect of human nature, leaders foster an environment where individuals have a sense of worth and understanding.

In contrast to prevailing perceptions, the integration of empathic leadership within the military domain does not entail a diminishment of discipline or a loosening of standards. Instead, it embodies a superior manifestation of leadership rooted in emotional intelligence. Achieving a calibrated equilibrium between a mission's imperatives and subordinates' well-being is imperative. The leader is compelled to make prudent decisions that encompass strategic factors and the inherent human elements that are invariably involved.

The significance of empathic leadership is derived from the fundamental role of the human factor in military undertakings. An army operation's effectiveness depends on the individuals responsible for carrying it out. In the present context, leadership is beyond the conventional notions of exercising authority and directing subordinates, as it encompasses the capacity to establish meaningful connections, understand diverse perspectives, and attentively consider the opinions and insights of people under one's guidance. The presence of empathy is crucial in facilitating these connections.

In addition, the use of empathetic leadership practices serves to bolster transparent communication, foster the development of trust, and strengthen the overall cohesiveness of teams. The resource in question plays a crucial role in conflict resolution, is of utmost importance in managing crises, and is a catalyst for fostering innovative problem-solving approaches. It effectively enhances the human aspect of military leadership, increasing its effectiveness in tangible ways.

Despite possessing formidable weaponry and employing complicated techniques, the military remains an institution ultimately composed of human beings. The concept of empathy acknowledges this indisputable reality and establishes it as a fundamental element of successful leadership. The prevailing perception of the stoic and autocratic leader is challenged and replaced by a paradigm emphasizing the need for emotional intelligence and a sophisticated comprehension of human behavior. Contrary to indicating a lack of strength, empathic leadership shows the leader's resilience, demonstrating their capacity to guide through intellectual prowess and emotional intelligence. The humanization of the military institution is paramount, as it strengthens intra-team relationships and bolsters the overall efficacy of leadership.

CHAPTER 3

THE MILITARY PARADIGM: FROM POWER TO EMPATHY

The traditional conception of the military leader as a resolute, stern authority figure is enduring a significant transformation. This change implies an essential shift in our perception of what military management entails; it is not only aesthetic. Military leaders have traditionally been held up as models of discipline and toughness, demonstrating qualities like bravery, decisiveness, and steadfast concentration. Although these qualities are still crucial, more people realize they are insufficient. Consequently, empathy is becoming an equally essential attribute for effective military leadership, a shift that challenges established norms and encourages a more nuanced and humane approach to command.

This transformation is anything but trivial; it represents a fundamental reevaluation of the framework in which we view military authority. Military institutions have historically favored leadership philosophies that emphasized conformity and obedience over the person's mental health. These institutions have traditionally relied on rigid codes of behavior and hierarchical organizational structures. According to a growing body of corporate behavior and psychology studies, the efficacy, team spirit, and resilience of an organization can all be improved by empathizing with others.

The importance of these benefits cannot be emphasized in the high-stakes setting of military activities, where lives frequently fall in danger. In order to improve communication, make more informed decisions, and take a more nuanced stance regarding the inevitable difficulties that develop in the extreme conditions of military conflicts, an empathic leader is more capable of gauging the psychological and mental well-being of their subordinates. They recognize that beneath the rigid structure of ranks and uniforms are individuals with anxieties, aspirations, and vulnerabilities.

The transition towards empathic leadership represents more than a mere softening of military power; rather, it signifies an expansion of its scope and approach. By integrating empathy into their leadership approaches, military leaders acquire a comprehensive comprehension of their personnel, which proves to be of immense value in both training exercises and actual operational contexts. These leaders are not forsaking the fundamental components of military command, namely discipline, strategic competence, and courage. Rather, they are enhancing these characteristics by incorporating a profound understanding of the human condition. It is acknowledged that military operations encompass more than just machinery and strategic planning, since they are intricately intertwined with human elements such as morale, stress, and collaboration.

Incorporating empathy into the repertoire of military leadership strategies presents novel opportunities for fostering enhanced interpersonal relationships, encompassing hierarchical connections among different levels and lateral bonds among colleagues. Encouraging open communication within a team environment promotes trust and contributes to developing a more robust and resilient team. Significantly, it serves to humanize a climate that frequently lacks humanity, allowing for the consideration of service members' emotional and psychological welfare, which is equally vital for achieving mission objectives as any strategic move.

The increasing acknowledgment of empathy's significance in military leadership signifies a significant transformation in cultural norms and operational tactics. The abovementioned change entails more than simply incorporating an additional ability into the repertoire of leadership abilities. Instead, it necessitates a profound reconsideration of strategies for fostering cultures that value authority and emotional intelligence. This transformative phenomenon holds the potential to not only redefine the essence of military leadership but also significantly impact future military operations' trajectory.

The False Dichotomy of Power and Empathy
The traditional perspective on military leadership, which prioritizes rigorous hierarchies, unshakable discipline, and inflexible regulations, has frequently been seen as inherently incompatible with the notion of empathy. This interpretation has given rise to the erroneous notion that military leaders have a binary choice between exercising authority and demonstrating compassion, as if both attributes cannot coexist. Nevertheless, the current comprehension of leadership dynamics is starting to question this presumption, proposing a significantly more comprehensive and mutually beneficial connection between power and empathy.

In this refined conceptual framework, the utilization of power through the perspective of empathy does not undermine the legitimacy or efficacy of a military commander. In contrast, it enhances said power's influence, increasing its effectiveness in cultivating allegiance, nurturing confidence, and establishing a unified entity. Leader who possesses empathy can effectively maneuver the intricate emotional terrain of their subordinates, augmenting their ability to make discerning decisions that consider not only strategic goals but also the human elements involved. Including this additional complexity allows for a more profound level of engagement with fellow team members, enhancing communication effectiveness, promoting seamless operational processes, and increasing the probability of achieving mission objectives.

Consider, for instance, the hypothetical situation of a platoon leader serving in the United States Army and deployed on a challenging international mission. The person under consideration, henceforth designated as Captain Smith, undertakes the responsibility of leading his men in challenging and arduous situations. A traditional, hierarchical approach may dictate that an individual issue commands without considering the emotional or psychological consequences on their subordinates, focusing solely on achieving the immediate goal.

In contrast, Captain Smith adopts a divergent methodology. The individual incorporates empathy into their leadership approach, acknowledging the significance of attuning to the cognitive and affective conditions of their subordinates. Prior to a crucial undertaking, the individual in question engages in concise one-on-one dialogues with his subordinates, whereby he acknowledges their apprehensions and unease, while also reiterating the inherent fortitude he perceives inside each of them. Engaging in this activity should not be perceived as a display of vulnerability or an inefficient utilization of valuable time. Instead, it should be regarded as a deliberate maneuver aimed at strengthening the psychological endurance of the collective group.

Upon encountering an unforeseen difficulty throughout the operation, the platoon has an increased propensity for open communication, as they possess a heightened level of faith in the value placed upon their contributions instead of being disregarded. This enables Captain Smith to make a judicious decision that not only overcomes the impediment but also safeguards the welfare of his troops. The task has been effectively accomplished, and it is equally significant to note that the warriors have a sense of recognition, attentiveness, and worth. Individuals who have experienced a leader who demonstrates understanding and concern toward them feel a sense of success and exhibit heightened loyalty and respect upon their return.

The compassionate leadership demonstrated by Captain Smith enhances his authority rather than diminishing it. The individual effectively utilizes the improved understanding and emotional connection provided by empathy to establish a more cohesive and resilient team, enhancing their ability to address the many obstacles encountered in contemporary combat effectively.

Hence, it may be argued that the conventional dichotomy juxtaposing authority and empathy is deceptive and undermines effectiveness. A more informed viewpoint suggests that instead of being in opposition to authority, the heart contributes to its improvement by adding a profound and intricate dimension that cultivates a more efficient and humane military leadership paradigm.

Power Reinvented through Empathy

The enduring principles of military leadership, including discipline, courage, and strategic intelligence, remain relevant in contemporary times. The aforementioned fundamental principles are not only essential but also necessary for the efficient execution of any military endeavor. However, it is imperative to comprehend that integrating empathy into leadership does not weaken these fundamental components; instead, it significantly enhances and magnifies them.

Consider, for example, the notion of discipline, a fundamental element within the military mentality. When disciplinary actions are administered without considering individual circumstances or demonstrating understanding, they can be readily seen as primarily punitive, as a means of exerting power and control. Nevertheless, when a leader adopts an empathetic perspective toward discipline, there is a notable transformation in the dynamics. Within this particular framework, discipline is applied with a comprehensive comprehension of the distinct requirements, encounters, and incentives of every individual within the team. Consequently, implementing disciplinary measures transforms into a platform for communal development rather than serving as a mechanism for individual retribution. The primary shift is observed in the transformation of emphasis from a hierarchical framework of punitive measures to a more egalitarian societal structure characterized by collective accountability and reciprocal regard.

As an illustration, let us consider the scenario with Commander Johnson, a U.S. Navy officer, and Petty Officer Williams, who serves as their subordinate. Consider a hypothetical scenario wherein Petty Officer Williams commits a transgression of a somewhat inconsequential yet significant rule about the appropriate storage of equipment while serving on a vessel. In a conventional disciplinary framework characterized by hierarchical power dynamics, Commander Johnson may promptly administer a reprimand or punitive action without comprehending the contextual factors or underlying motivations that led to the transgression.

Nevertheless, Commander Johnson opts for another course of action. Acknowledging the significance of empathy in the realm of effective leadership, she initiates a private conversation with Williams to comprehend the underlying reasons behind the occurrence of the mistake. During their dialogue, she learned that Williams needed more clarity on the recently introduced storage standards. Rather than administering a formal reprimand, Commander Johnson seizes this opportunity to provide a valuable lesson to Williams and the entire squad. The individual arranges a training session to elucidate the recently established protocols, guaranteeing a shared understanding among all participants.

What is the outcome? Williams expresses gratitude for the opportunity to acquire knowledge and enhance skills rather than experiencing a sense of discouragement due to punitive measures. The implementation of renewed training has a positive impact on the entire team, decreasing the probability of recurring errors in subsequent instances. Significantly, the culture on the ship undergoes a subtle yet perceptible transformation, characterized by a collective sense of responsibility and mutual regard. These outcomes can be attributed to applying discipline incorporating empathy and a comprehensive grasp of the human context.

Fundamentally, the authority possessed by Commander Johnson, when combined with empathy, transformed a crude mechanism utilized to exert control into a sophisticated instrument that improved the overall welfare of her military unit. The transformation of discipline occurred as it shifted from a tool of intimidation to a means of fostering personal development, strengthening the connections of trust and admiration within the team. Hence, it may be argued that empathy does not supplant the fundamental tenets of military leadership; instead, it imbues them with enhanced profundity and scope, engendering a more efficacious and human-centered paradigm for contemporary military operations.

The Transformation: A Journey, not a Destination

Shifting from a leadership model that only focused on exerting power to one that effectively integrates empathy is a gradual and challenging endeavor. The process of this transformation is deliberate and requires consistent dedication and a reassessment of deeply rooted norms and habits. The process involves a transformation in cognitive perspective and a progressive enhancement in how military commanders perceive and understand their responsibilities, duties, and interactions within the hierarchical framework. The antiquated framework that previously defined military leadership exclusively regarding command, control, and coercion is gradually diminishing. A novel paradigm is currently being observed: the leader embodying the role of an "empathetic guide." This individual not only prioritizes the attainment of strategic goals but also demonstrates a profound commitment to their staff's emotional and psychological welfare.

Major Smith, a battalion commander within the United States Army, initially adopted a conventional leadership approach characterized by a strong emphasis on rules, commands, and discipline. The efficacy of his leadership style could have been improved insofar as it facilitated the efficient functioning of activities yet inadvertently hindered individual initiative and impeded the free flow of communication among subordinates. Service Members frequently show reluctance in expressing their opinions or concerns, primarily due to apprehension regarding potential censure or dismissal. In summary, Major Smith held a position of authority, yet he needed a genuine rapport with his subordinates.

Acknowledging his methodology's constraints, Major Smith committed to adapting and developing his technique. The individual commenced attending seminars centered around empathic leadership and engaged in significant reading on emotional intelligence. However, of utmost significance, he initiated the implementation of incremental and regular modifications in his engagements with his staff. Instead of solely giving directives, he initiated the practice of soliciting comments. Instead of simply demanding obedience, he fostered debates that facilitated nuanced comprehension of intricate circumstances. The individual initiated a systematic implementation of morale assessments and established mechanisms for anonymous input to assess the emotional atmosphere inside his battalion.

During a specific occurrence, the battalion encountered a notably demanding field exercise. Instead of resorting to his previous authoritarian methods, Major Smith utilized his recently acquired sympathetic abilities. The individual in question solicited feedback from his subordinates regarding the most effective approach to managing the intricate situation, integrating their perspectives into the ultimate strategic plan. Furthermore, acknowledging the inherently demanding character of the activity, he orchestrated a post-event evaluation that encompassed a strategic examination and a dialogue regarding the team's emotional response to the encounter.

The outcomes exhibited a significant transforming effect. The battalion achieved success in their field exercise and demonstrated an enhanced level of group ownership and morale. The attitude of Major Smith underwent a subtle yet substantial transformation, transitioning from a predominantly authoritative style to one that integrated elements of authority, empathy, and inclusiveness.

The journey undertaken by Major Smith serves as a poignant illustration of the gradual yet significant transition from a power-focused paradigm to one that prioritizes empathy. The individual in question did not relinquish his position of authority or forsake the fundamental tenets of military leadership. Conversely, he augmented their comprehension by imparting an extra stratum of human insight, transforming his position from an authoritative leader to a compassionate mentor. Major Smith successfully achieved his strategic objectives through this action while cultivating a stronger, more robust, and ultimately more efficient combat unit.

The Human Element: Recognizing Individuality

Recognizing the inherent individuality of service members, characterized by their distinct attributes, competencies, aspirations, and anxieties, holds paramount significance for any proficient military leader. Failure to acknowledge this essential comprehension can lead to a uniform approach to leadership, which not only hampers personal uniqueness but also fosters a constricting atmosphere. In a setting of this nature, commands can be carried out without being internalized. Respect may appear to be present on the surface, as it is enforced through hierarchical positions. Still, it may not be legitimately earned through the establishment of mutual trust and understanding. Recognizing the distinctiveness of every service member facilitates a customized and intricate method of leadership, which not only upholds the integrity of each soldier but also maximizes their capabilities, thus enhancing the overall efficiency and unity of the entire unit.

Lieutenant Johnson was an officer serving as a platoon leader within the United States Marine Corps. At the outset, the man in question perceived his platoon as a homogeneous entity, a cohesive unit that necessitated synchronized movement and action, with limited consideration for individual differences. The lack of attention to this matter decreased morale and suboptimal performance during training activities. Nevertheless, upon recognizing this pattern, Lieutenant Johnson decided to allocate his time to engaging in individualized conversations to develop a deeper understanding of each member of his platoon.

During these interpersonal exchanges, it was ascertained that Corporal Martinez possessed exceptional proficiency in marksmanship, with a profound inclination towards data analytics. However, it was seen that his enthusiasm towards physical training was comparatively less pronounced. Conversely, Sergeant Williams had exceptional proficiency in physical agility, although they exhibited relatively lower levels of involvement in planning and strategy. Acknowledging these distinctive characteristics, Lieutenant Johnson redistributed duties in a manner that capitalized on his team's individual abilities. Corporal Martinez was assigned a multifaceted task that integrated his proficiency in marksmanship with data analysis during reconnaissance missions. Sergeant Williams assumed responsibility for conducting physical training sessions, infusing them with unparalleled enthusiasm derived from his innate athleticism.

This alteration yielded several advantages. Initially, every individual within the group experienced a sense of worth and comprehension, resulting in a noticeable enhancement in overall morale. Furthermore, via the strategic assignment of activities aligned with each member's unique abilities and interests, Lieutenant Johnson observed a significant increase in levels of engagement and commitment. The nature of orders transformed from mere directives to be followed to meaningful missions that elicited personal promises from every individual involved. Finally, the admiration for Lieutenant Johnson increased, not alone due to his position, but as evidence of his capacity to comprehend and proficiently guide his crew.

The comprehension of individuality does not undermine the hierarchical structure but enhances it. This capability enables the leader to leverage the vast array of abilities and motivations inside the unit, transforming a homogeneous group of troops into a versatile and dynamic team capable of effectively responding to various problems. The narrative of Lieutenant Johnson serves as an illustrative example that highlights the potential advantages of acknowledging and valuing the distinctiveness of individuals within a military organization. This case study demonstrates how adopting such an approach imbues the hierarchical structure with a sense of humanity and enhances its overall efficacy.

The Practical Implications: Building Stronger Units
The utilization of empathetic leadership extends beyond the mere process of humanizing the military setting. It possesses practical and mission-critical ramifications that have the potential to determine the success or failure of operations. A leader who possesses empathy is equipped with the necessary abilities to mitigate internal tensions and effectively address issues in an advantageous manner to all individuals involved. A leader of this nature establishes a conducive climate where open communication is not only endorsed but also essential for the effective operation of the group. In this particular context, the decision-making process becomes more inclusive and insightful. The willingness of team members to communicate their views, concerns, and suggestions contributes to a more comprehensive grasp of the current situation. Consequently, this provides the leader with diverse perspectives necessary for enhanced strategy planning and implementation. Developing and maintaining a bond based on respect and mutual trust can significantly impact the result, determining success or failure, in situations marked by significant stakes and mission-criticality.

Captain Smith, an officer serving as a company commander within the United States Army, was responsible for managing a complex counter-insurgency campaign. The mission was characterized by intricate challenges pertaining to civilian populations, antagonistic rebels, and hazardous topography. In the first stages, Captain Smith employed a hierarchical strategy wherein he did not actively pursue or place importance on soliciting feedback from his subordinates. The outcome entailed a sequence of errors that not only jeopardized the successful execution of the operation but also contributed to escalating tensions inside the unit.

Acknowledging the significance of the circumstances and the declining morale, Captain Smith decided to transition towards a leadership approach characterized by more empathy. The individual initiated the process by organizing open forums where team members were encouraged to express their viewpoints regarding the challenges encountered and propose potential adaptations. Specialist Brown, an adept soldier with prior experience in urban fighting, proposed modifying their patrol patterns, drawing upon his knowledge of local cultural norms. This adjustment has the potential to render their movements less foreseeable to insurgents.

In light of the valuable insights provided by Specialist Brown, Captain Smith made necessary modifications to the operational plan. The newly implemented strategy demonstrated enhanced efficacy and instilled within the team a renewed sense of ownership toward the purpose. The individuals experienced a feeling of being acknowledged and appreciated, enhancing their confidence in the leadership abilities of Captain Smith. Upon encountering a precarious circumstance with potential mortal consequences, the presence of mutual respect and open communication among the individuals involved expedited and enabled prompt and efficient measures, ultimately culminating in the triumph of the mission.

The entirety of the story provided a clear and compelling demonstration of the tangible advantages associated with leadership that are characterized by empathy. Through establishing effective communication channels and recognizing subordinate information, Captain Smith successfully acquired a broader spectrum of perspectives to inform his decision-making process. Furthermore, the trust and respect he garnered from his team proved to be a tremendous asset in the demanding and unpredictable circumstances frequently encountered in military endeavors.

In brief, the practice of empathic leadership not only fosters a more amicable work atmosphere but also significantly enhances the efficacy and accomplishments of the organizational unit. Cultivating trust and open communication can significantly influence the outcomes of the intricate and demanding circumstances frequently encountered by military forces. The experience of Captain Smith provides a valuable case study that highlights the significance of empathy in leadership, emphasizing that it is not merely a desirable quality but rather an essential asset crucial to the success of a mission.

Resilience Through Empathy

The relevance of empathic leadership is magnified when considering the severe conditions and high-stress environments prevalent in military operations. A leader who possesses a profound understanding of their employees exhibits enhanced effectiveness in their day-to-day leadership and plays a significant role in bolstering the unit's resilience when confronted with adversities. In situations that require considerable physical exertion or involve high emotional strain, such as prolonged deployments, combat scenarios, or disaster relief operations, the ability of a compassionate leader to identify early indicators of stress, exhaustion, or mental distress can be of great importance. By rapidly detecting these difficulties, leaders can respond before escalating into more severe problems such as physical injuries or mental health crises. Using a proactive approach contributes to the sustained operational readiness of the unit in the long run and can potentially mitigate potential loss of life.

Lieutenant Johnson assumed the role of commanding officer for a United States Marine Corps battalion during a prolonged international mission. Recognizing the potential adverse effects on both physical and psychological health resulting from such deployments, Johnson adopted a proactive stance in safeguarding the overall welfare of his unit. The individual consistently engaged in periodic assessments with team members, employing both structured and unstructured approaches, fostering an environment conducive to Marines expressing their apprehensions or challenges without hesitation. During one of these routine assessments, Johnson saw that Corporal Williams, a typically optimistic and proficient Marine, exhibited uncharacteristic reticence and manifested minor indications of physical exhaustion.

In light of perceiving the initial indicators, Lieutenant Johnson conducted a more comprehensive investigation. During an individualized dialogue, it was established that Williams was experiencing sleep deprivation due to operational stress and personal concerns in his domestic environment. Instead of disregarding it as a predictable aspect of military existence or perceiving it as vulnerability, Johnson recognized the issue and promptly implemented measures to address it. The job roster of Corporal Williams was modified to accommodate additional periods of respite, and arrangements were made for him to engage in a consultation with a mental health professional inside the military.

The intervention yielded a dual outcome, as it facilitated Corporal Williams in obtaining the necessary rest and support, thereby enhancing his operational efficacy. Furthermore, this action effectively conveyed a significant message to the remaining members of the unit, indicating that their leader possessed a genuine and sincere interest in their welfare. Consequently, it fostered an environment where seeking assistance when necessary was deemed acceptable. This facilitated a conducive atmosphere characterized by trust and transparency, hence enhancing the overall resilience of the unit. Over the course of its existence, the unit has constantly garnered recognition for its exceptional operational readiness and minimal incidence of burnout or other stress-related problems. This serves as a testimonial to the significance of employing empathic leadership inside the organization.

Lieutenant Johnson's approach exemplifies the actual application of empathic leadership, showcasing its profound impact on bolstering the resilience of a military force. Through the identification of first indicators of stress and exhaustion and the prompt implementation of appropriate measures, Johnson effectively averted the risk of burnout for a crucial member of the team, while simultaneously fostering a culture that promotes the enduring well-being and productivity of the entire unit. In essence, this exemplifies the efficacy of empathetic leadership, wherein empathy is transformed from a non-technical skill into a strategic resource.

In contrast to certain existing perspectives, it is argued that a military leader who demonstrates empathy should not be perceived as a "weak" leader. On the contrary, a leader of this nature possesses the resilience to comprehend the intricacies of human emotions and situations, and to approach them in a productive fashion. The leadership style exhibited by the individual in question surpasses traditional boundaries of authority, establishing a connection with the profound aspects of shared human experiences. The utilization of a comprehensive strategy in leadership incorporates the integration of emotional intelligence and rational cognition, leading to a military unit that demonstrates enhanced efficiency and unity, while also exhibiting a deep understanding of its own human nature.

CHAPTER 4

SHIFTING PERSPECTIVES: EMPATHY IN TRAINING

For a sizable amount of time, it has been known that military instruction and the growth of warriors are related. The ability to tolerate and overcome great barriers and the resolve to persevere in the face of difficulty are qualities that this training is renowned to inculcate and foster. These qualities are essential to the identification of a warrior. The primary objective has consistently been cultivating resilience, discipline, and a combined physical and mental fortitude. The ideas above, which have been transmitted across successive generations, constitute the fundamental basis of the military ethos.

Nevertheless, our comprehension of the qualities that constitute a genuinely proficient military leader transforms as time progresses. One characteristic that may initially appear incongruous within this particular environment is empathy. The intense standards of military training are not typically associated with this specific quality.

However, the importance of this cannot be exaggerated. When leaders fail to establish a meaningful connection and understanding of their subordinates' lived experiences, their leadership effectiveness diminishes. Without empathy, the capacity to cultivate team cohesion reduces, compromising the ability to effectively utilize a group's collective skills and abilities. The significance of empathy in the contemporary military environment becomes evident.

Integrating empathy into military training does not compromise the intensity or intensity of the routine. In contrast, it expands its scope, extending the instruction to encompass a more comprehensive perspective. Engaging in this practice enhances the underlying framework on which military members are constructed, guaranteeing their emotional resilience is on par with their physical strength.

One notable facet of this revised strategy entails the

inclusion of training modules that emphasize the development of emotional intelligence. These modules consist of activities designed to enhance self-awareness, promote a more comprehensive comprehension of varied perspectives, and cultivate stronger emotional connections among members of a team. Consider it as the provision of service members with instruments that guarantee their continuous awareness of both their external environment and their own emotional states, as well as those of their fellow service members.

For example, one may examine the potential benefits of including team-building activities within boot camp programs. Rather than exclusively emphasizing arduous physical tasks, the curriculum has the potential to integrate role-playing exercises. These workshops would provide participants with immersive experiences that facilitate their understanding of the diverse emotional states and external stressors that service member may encounter while in active service.

Taking an additional stride, envision the profound impact that including regular mindfulness sessions in a soldier's regimen could have. The use of this technique, which focuses on the improvement of emotional consciousness, would be equally crucial to any strategic exercise. Ultimately, the ability to comprehend and manage one's own emotions, as well as the emotions of others, can significantly impact the efficacy of decision-making in circumstances characterized by intense stress.

The effort to incorporate empathy into training necessitates a novel approach to evaluating and quantifying achievement inside the military hierarchy. Historically, assessments have been based on objective and well-defined standards, such as mastery of particular competencies or the capacity to endure physically demanding activities.

Nevertheless, the emerging perspective proposes that these indicators, although still crucial, must be more isolated. There is a growing recognition that incorporating measurements pertaining to emotional intelligence is becoming increasingly important and should be integrated with traditional benchmarks. Military training has the potential to cultivate a holistic comprehension of a soldier's aptitudes, encompassing their physical and emotional capacities.

Let us contemplate the consequences ensuing from a simulated military conflict exercise. In this advanced training concept, debriefings would encompass a more comprehensive examination beyond the conventional tactical analysis. In addition to analyzing the employed tactics and evaluating their efficacy, these sessions would also address the scenario's emotional dynamics. Conversations may shift towards identifying instances characterized by heightened terror, evaluating the approaches employed to manage such situations, and exploring alternative emotional methods. Implementing a tiered strategy guarantees that service members' emotional well-being and resilience are accorded equal significance to their tactical proficiency.

The narrative of Captain Smith is a captivating account. Upon assuming the leadership role of a specialist military unit, Captain Smith was confronted with the task of supervising a rigorous training regimen. The primary objective of this program was not just to provide his squad with the necessary skills for routine drills but rather to adequately train them for highly demanding overseas operations.

Smith's routine was enhanced by introducing a novel element, "empathy circles," which acknowledged a sometimes disregarded facet. The individual comprehended the significance of emotional intelligence in cultivating robust and resilient teams. During these sessions, he motivated team members to openly discuss their experiences, express their most urgent issues, and communicate their objectives.

The outcomes were undeniably revolutionary. An unforeseen advantage was uncovered upon deployment of the unit in a high-risk operational environment characterized by elevated stress levels. The emotional connections they had established and cultivated throughout their training now served as a source of unspoken resilience. Establishing these deep ties resulted in improved interpersonal communication, expedited decision-making processes, and cultivated a sense of cohesion among individuals. Ultimately, the cohesive camaraderie and mutual comprehension exhibited by the individuals involved proved to be not only advantageous but also pivotal in achieving resounding triumph in their goal.

Through this approach, the traditional military training is not being diluted, but rather enhanced. The physical exercises, cognitive demands, and strategic teachings all remain unchanged. Nevertheless, a notable alteration lies in integrating a crucial novel component, namely empathy, intricately interwoven like a precious thread inside the framework of military readiness.

In this immersive training environment, the emerging military personnel are being prepared for a range of skills beyond tactical proficiency and physical endurance. This establishment's educational program and guiding principles are designed to cultivate well-rounded leaders who can lead effectively in both practical and emotionally intelligent ways.

The military establishment has concluded that authentic

strength encompasses various dimensions. It is not exclusively derived from physical strength or strategic intelligence.

Moreover, emotional adaptability plays a vital role in navigating the intricate web of human interactions, particularly under demanding circumstances where each choice has substantial consequences.

We are leaving behind established, conventional power systems as we embark on this historic transformation. Instead, we are embracing a fresh inquiry style grounded in compassion and comprehension. This represents a significant shift in the way leadership is understood and practiced.

Empathy is no longer a byproduct or an afterthought in this more advanced way of teaching service members. It is being put in the spotlight and made a regular part of the training that is just as important as any tactical skill or physical regimen.

Empathy is no longer seen as a possible weakness or flaw. Instead, it symbolizes strength and a key part of modern, changing military training, leadership, and general philosophy.

CHAPTER 5

FROM BOOTS TO HEART: NURTURING EMOTIONAL INTELLIGENCE

When contemplating the military, one's thoughts are often inundated with a series of vivid mental images akin to a meticulously curated compilation of precisely synchronized footsteps of impeccably polished boots, immaculate uniforms embellished with resplendent medals that recount tales of bravery, and a discernible atmosphere of resolute discipline that can almost be felt. Within our observations, there exist specific individuals who exemplify the highest level of physical strength and strategic acumen. These individuals undergo rigorous training not only in the mastery of weaponry but also in the intricate principles and tactics of warfare. The shown image is a captivating representation that is deeply rooted in long-standing traditions and cultural veneration. It prominently highlights attributes such as discipline, physical prowess, and strategic intelligence. Nevertheless, a notable omission in this widely acknowledged account is the significance of emotional intelligence.

In an environment characterized by situations of significant stress, high stakes, and considerable uncertainty, where decisions can have life-or-death consequences, the ability to comprehend, regulate, and skillfully employ emotions emerges as a crucial form of expertise, comparable in importance to proficiency in handling firearms or devising offensive strategies. Emotional intelligence holds significant importance and should not be regarded as a peripheral or discretionary attribute that leaders can disregard. Establishing a coherent entity capable of operating at peak efficiency even in the most challenging circumstances is of utmost importance. Gaining insight into the methods of motivating a varied range of persons, each with distinct psychological compositions and emotional requirements, is paramount when striving to achieve a shared goal under challenging conditions.

Moreover, the concept of emotional intelligence enables

leaders to enhance their self-awareness by recognizing their personal biases, effectively managing their stress levels, making well-rounded decisions, and, significantly, establishing empathetic connections with their subordinates. A leader's capacity to demonstrate empathy towards their team members contributes to establishing trust and promoting reciprocal respect that cannot be achieved solely through hierarchical positions. The comprehensive military leader is, therefore, not only a strategist or an enforcer but also a scholar of humanities, demonstrating acute sensitivity towards the emotional dynamics that exist both within their own persona and among their subordinates.

When considering the attributes that characterize a prosperous military leader, adopting a more comprehensive perspective is imperative. In addition to the requisite tactical skills and physical stamina, it is essential to consider the inclusion of emotional understanding and sympathetic wisdom as crucial factors that distinguish competent leaders from exceptional ones. Emotional intelligence should not be viewed as the opposite of military toughness but rather as a complementary trait. In a domain that necessitates the possession of both martial valor and intellectual wisdom, the significance of emotional intelligence transcends mere importance and assumes a position of utmost necessity.

Consider a hypothetical scenario whereby a platoon leader has exceptional proficiency in executing tactical actions while simultaneously exhibiting the ability to discern the morale of their subordinates. An effective leader possesses the ability to discern when a team member is experiencing difficulties without overt communication and may offer empathetic support without verbal expression. This leader demonstrates expertise not only in strategic warfare but also in the cultivation of empathy. The individuals comprehend that effective leadership encompasses both emotional intelligence and authoritative control.

The cultivation of emotional intelligence inside the military is initiated by acknowledging its inherent worth. Understanding that it is a crucial component of it is important rather than considering the capacity for greater human understanding as generally going against military might. People with a high ability to comprehend people more profoundly can grasp, use, and positively control their sentiments to reduce stress, advance viable correspondence, demonstrate sympathy for others, overcome challenges, and resolve concerns. The concept extends beyond mere subjective experience of emotions, encompassing their utilization to gain deeper comprehension, make more informed choices, and exhibit superior leadership skills.

The development of emotional intelligence includes several key components, including the development of a sense of emotion, the use of emotions, and the control of emotions. We shall continue to dissect the issue at hand in this examination.

Emotional Awareness:
Emotional awareness, a fundamental aspect of emotional intelligence, pertains to the capacity to effectively recognize and comprehend not just one's own emotional states but also those shown by individuals in one's immediate environment. The process extends beyond identifying overt, vibrant displays, such as smiles or frowns. It encompasses the perception of more nuanced nonverbal signals, including vocal intonation, body position, and even ocular movements. Furthermore, emotional awareness encompasses the ability to comprehend the collective emotional climate inside a group or team context, facilitating the discernment of the presence of tension,

camaraderie, stress, or exhilaration.

The significance of emotional awareness in a military situation cannot be overemphasized. Consider the hypothetical scenario in which Lieutenant Johnson has the role of commanding a group of military personnel on a mission of great importance involving reconnaissance activities. Johnson observes that one of his crucial team members, Specialist Brown, exhibits signs of physical preparedness but displays a little deviation from his usual demeanor, possibly shown by mild strain in his shoulders or an abnormally somber tone of speech. Due to the significant importance of the mission, Johnson discreetly requests a private conversation with Brown, creating an environment conducive to open communication. During this exchange, Brown discloses that he has recently received distressing information from his personal life, which could potentially impact his ability to concentrate on the task at hand.

Rather than disregarding these emotional signals or merely expecting an unyielding display of stoicism, Johnson employs his emotional intelligence to comprehend the emotional condition of his team member. The individual in question may opt to redistribute certain responsibilities assigned to Brown for the mission among other members of the team, while concurrently offering more emotional support to aid in his coping process, all while maintaining the integrity of the mission's objectives. This action not only preserves unit cohesion but also amplifies it. Through the act of recognizing and attending to Brown's emotional condition, Johnson cultivates an environment characterized by trust and mutual regard. Currently, each member of the team possesses an understanding that their worth extends beyond their functional responsibilities. They recognize that their leader is attentive to their overall welfare, rather than solely focusing on their specific skill set.

Therefore, the cultivation of emotional awareness transcends being merely a soft talent and instead assumes a crucial role as an essential operational tool. The utilization of this approach empowers military commanders to make well-informed judgments that effectively balance the tactical imperatives with the emotional and psychological welfare of the personnel, thereby augmenting the overall effectiveness of the unit and the successful accomplishment of the mission.

Emotional Application

The utilization of emotional intelligence extends beyond mere recognition and comprehension of emotions. It encompasses the application of emotional intelligence as a practical instrument to direct behaviors, decision-making, and interpersonal engagements. This entails utilizing one's understanding of personal and interpersonal emotional states to proficiently address challenges, devise strategies, and facilitate enhanced communication within a team. This attribute should not be seen solely as an abstract "soft skill," but rather as a pivotal element that has the potential to determine the outcome of both individual and collaborative undertakings.

Consider the case of Captain Smith, who is now overseeing her squad as they engage in a rigorous and demanding simulation aimed at equipping them with the necessary skills and readiness for actual combat situations. During a period of heightened emotions, she observes an increase in both tension and stress levels among her colleagues. This may be indicated by instances of irritability or a disruption in their typical patterns of communication. Utilizing her adeptness in emotional regulation, she not only discerns the escalation of stress levels but also devises prompt strategies to channel this emotional energy in a constructive manner.

Captain Smith convenes a prompt gathering and utilizes a stress management technique that she has acquired, leading her squad through a swift succession of deep-breathing exercises or a concise motivational discourse with the intention of redirecting their attention and revitalizing their energy. The individual possesses an understanding that stress encompasses more than simply a psychological condition, as it elicits physiological responses that can detrimentally influence one's performance, including but not limited to decision-making speed, concentration, and even motor abilities. Through the efficient application of her comprehension of emotions, she is not merely enhancing the overall emotional state, but rather directly augmenting the likelihood of accomplishing the task.

Moreover, it is possible that she could employ affective reasoning in the process of formulating strategies and making decisions. Given the awareness of her team's heightened stress levels, she can choose to employ a strategy that capitalizes on their individual strengths and preexisting skill sets, rather than implementing a novel and intricate plan that could potentially exacerbate their stress levels.

Captain Smith effectively utilizes emotional intelligence to inform her leadership decisions, hence enhancing the cohesion, effectiveness, and operational performance of the unit. The utilization of emotional application is a valuable asset within a leader's repertoire, as it possesses the ability to effectively respond to diverse circumstances and positively impact both the individual's welfare and the group's achievements.

Emotional Regulation

The ability to manage emotions is a crucial talent that

reaches beyond simple self-control. It involves a dynamic interaction between regulating one's own emotional state and exerting influence over the vibrant atmosphere within a collective, particularly in demanding and consequential settings such as the military. This necessitates adopting a comprehensive approach, encompassing the utilization of stress-management methodologies for individuals and implementing tactics that bolster team morale and foster unity. The value of creating an environment that supports everyone's maximum performance, especially in highly stressful situations, lies in addition to keeping composure.

Consider the situation of Sergeant Johnson, who takes charge of a specialized team tasked with eliminating improvised explosive devices (IEDs). The inherent characteristics of the occupation are profoundly demanding, as it involves the direct responsibility for preserving human lives. On a particular occasion, his military unit is summoned to a highly critical site where the absence of success is not a viable outcome. The atmosphere is charged with tension, with the younger soldiers displaying visible signs of anxiety.

Sergeant Johnson, in light of the significance of the circumstances and the psychological burden experienced by his squad, prioritizes the appropriate management of his own stress levels. The individual employs several strategies, like as concentrated breathing and positive visualization, which have been refined through extensive practice, in order to maintain a state of centeredness. By prioritizing the management of his own emotional state, he enhances his capacity to function as a calming force for his team. The individual's composed disposition is not merely a facade, but rather a deliberately nurtured emotional state that confers advantages onto those in his vicinity.

Subsequently, he proceeds to actively undertake measures

aimed at exerting influence over the emotional atmosphere within his unit. Instead of disregarding the conspicuous issue at hand, he acknowledges the psychological strain and significance of the circumstance, nevertheless presents it as a chance for the team to showcase their expertise and preparation. The individual in question may opt to employ a personal narrative or employ humor as a means to alleviate any prevailing tension, so establishing a sense of relatability and fostering a more approachable atmosphere in relation to the given task. Additionally, he might seize the opportunity to prompt individuals to reflect about their previous accomplishments and the comprehensive instruction they have received, quietly enhancing their self-assurance.

Sergeant Johnson may opt to assign less experienced soldiers to more seasoned team members, not alone for the purpose of acquiring technical skills, but also to benefit from the emotional support and stability that the veterans can offer. By implementing this approach, the individual establishes a setting characterized by reciprocal regard and reliance, a condition that has been empirically demonstrated to diminish stress levels and enhance overall performance.

Through the proficient management of emotions, encompassing both personal and team-related sentiments, Sergeant Johnson enhances the likelihood of accomplishing missions successfully, while concurrently fostering the enduring emotional welfare of his unit. The leader's demonstrated ability to effectively combine emotional intelligence with tactical expertise highlights the significance of emotional management as a crucial asset in contemporary military operations.

The inclusion of these components into military training programs has the potential to foster the development of emotional intelligence from its foundational stages. The objective can be facilitated by the provision of workshops focused on emotional awareness, team-building activities designed to foster emotional understanding, and stress management approaches aimed at improving emotional regulation.

The transition from focusing on physical strength to developing emotional intelligence is a gradual process that only occurs sometimes. The process necessitates dedication to altering perspectives, modifying training initiatives, and reevaluating criteria for measuring achievement. This process entails dismantling the barriers of emotional stoicism and constructing pathways for emotional connection.

It is important to note that fostering emotional intelligence within the military does not suggest a reduction in the significance of physical fitness, tactical proficiency, or strategic cognition. Contrarily, it augments these facets by including a level of emotional comprehension that strengthens the unity of a team, enhances the process of making decisions, and cultivates a leadership style characterized by compassion and empathy.

As we progress in our exploration of the transition from power to empathy, it is imperative that we prioritize the establishment of a frequently traversed route connecting the realm of action and authority to that of compassion and understanding. The proposal entails the establishment of a military culture that places significant emphasis on the recognition, cultivation, and commemoration of emotional intelligence. This entails acknowledging the equal importance of emotional intelligence alongside physical preparedness, and advocating for leaders who exhibit not only intellectual acumen but also emotional acuity.

CHAPTER 6

FROM BARRACKS TO BATTLEFIELD: EMPATHY IN ACTION

The experience of navigating military life provides a distinct context in which the concept of empathy can be translated from a theoretical comprehension to practical implementation. The various aspects and stages of military life, including the repetitive nature of daily activities in barracks and the intense and high-pressure environment of the battlefield, serve as significant opportunities for the cultivation and application of empathy. The difficulty lies not only in comprehending the potential coexistence of empathy, intellectual rigor, and practical skills, but also in effectively manifesting this integration in practice.

Within the confines of the regimented setting of the barracks, the concept of empathy may appear to be an abstract moral quality, yet its practical expressions are indeed discernible. The act of active participation goes beyond merely nodding compassionately. The act of attentively listening to a fellow soldier's concerns regarding an upcoming deployment, providing emotional support in times of distressing news from their home, or engaging in a moment of solace over a cup of coffee after a physically and mentally demanding day are all integral components that contribute to the formation of empathy.

This extends beyond the realm of team morale. The cultivation of empathy within military barracks plays a crucial role in achieving strategic objectives by strengthening the fundamental cohesion of the unit, so establishing a foundation for collective resilience and enhancing the overall efficacy of mission execution. A team characterized by the perception of each member being acknowledged, listened to, and appreciated is a team that possesses the ability to confront the most severe obstacles with an unwavering determination.

In the context of warfare, the manifestation of empathy undergoes alterations while its enduring nature remains unaltered. In the context of enormous stakes and potential life-altering consequences, the fundamental principles of compassionate leadership persist. The capacity to assess strategic benefits in relation to the tangible consequences on human lives. A leader who can anticipate and consider the emotional and psychological consequences of battle decisions exemplifies the pinnacle of empathy.

An illustrative case is that of Lieutenant James Carter, who was assigned the responsibility of commanding a perilous mission. Upon observing one of his subordinates displaying signs of worry and hesitation before entering a dangerous zone, Carter allocated a little time to address the concerned individual privately. Instead of reprimanding him for his fear, Carter acknowledged and expressed his own, instilling the soldier with the resolve to go. Subsequently, during the aforementioned military action, when the opposing combatants were apprehended, how they were handled adhered not only to the prescribed rules of engagement but also showed a notable degree of respect and consideration, significantly impacting the morale of Carter's own forces. He demonstrated that even amid the abhorrent acts committed during times of armed conflict, the capacity for human compassion and decency may ultimately triumph.

Operationalizing empathy encompasses a comprehensive dedication, spanning from the mundane aspects of daily life within the barracks to the significant and transformative occurrences experienced on the battlefield. There is a need to integrate empathy deeply into the fundamental elements of military culture, ensuring its presence is as tangible as the physical sensations of holding a rifle or wearing a uniform. This statement shows the simultaneous presence of bravery and empathy, self-control and comprehension, and leadership and modesty.

In conclusion, it may be argued that empathy should not be

regarded as a passive characteristic. The incorporation of this dynamic, resilient, and transformative entity into the military ethos is both imperative and opportune. As we traverse the dynamic landscape of empathetic leadership within the military, it is imperative that we advocate for empathy not merely as a passive concept, but rather as an active guiding principle. This approach aims to reconcile the dichotomies that exist between the cognitive and affective aspects, the hierarchical and communal dynamics, and the contrasting forces of aggression and compassion, in order to establish a more comprehensive and compassionate framework for military duty.

CHAPTER 7

THE EMPATHY RIPPLE EFFECT: FROM LEADERSHIP TO CULTURE TRANSFORMATION

Leadership is frequently viewed as a prominent symbol, serving as a centralized source of direction and power. Nevertheless, a more intricate depiction emerges with a closer examination of empathic leadership. One may envision a pebble being cast into a serene lake, resulting in ripples that propagate outward, exerting influence upon all entities they come into contact with. The phenomenon referred to as the "Empathy Ripple Effect" exemplifies the influential role of an empathetic leader in cultivating a culture of empathy among team members.

The initiation of this ripple effect can be traced back to the individual in a position of leadership. A leader who possesses a high level of emotional attunement assumes a central role in driving the empathic movement. A leader of this nature cultivates an environment that places importance on emotional intelligence, wherein emotions are not merely accepted but embraced, and personal difficulties are not disregarded but actively confronted.

The initial wave originates from individuals in close proximity to the leader, such as subordinates, aides, or even peer officers. The aforementioned individuals are the initial recipients of the advantages derived from the leader's emotional intelligence. The researchers note the leader's astute comprehension of human emotions, their ability to acknowledge and affirm various viewpoints, and their authentic commitment to the welfare of others. As the level of appreciation and comprehension towards these intimate connections grows, people also take a more compassionate stance, hence intensifying the initial ripple effect.

An illustrative case is that of Captain Sarah Williams, who assumed command of a military unit characterized by elevated levels of stress and diminished morale. From the first, she made a firm commitment to implementing an open-door policy in principle and practical application, thereby ensuring her accessibility and attentiveness. In a situation where one of her subordinates was experiencing personal difficulties that had a negative impact on his job performance, rather than resorting to disciplinary measures, she opted to provide support by encouraging him to openly discuss his troubles and facilitating his access to appropriate professional resources. The sergeant demonstrated notable improvement and assumed the role of a loud proponent for mental health assistance inside the unit, amplifying the diffusion of empathy to a greater extent.

As the diffusion of empathy culture occurs through emulation and experiential learning, its effects become perceptible even among individuals who have limited direct engagement with the leader. The alteration of the team environment induces modifications in the chemistry, thereby stimulating open and honest communication, establishing a foundation of trust, and cultivating a feeling of interdependence. Over time, empathy evolves from a learned behavior to a highly esteemed cultural standard, deeply embedded within team dynamics, decision-making structures, and even approaches to resolving conflicts.

Sustaining this ripple of empathy requires continuous and deliberate effort rather than occurring automatically. Leaders must exemplify empathy consistently, provide training programs that cultivate emotional intelligence, and integrate these empathetic norms into the unit's foundational values. Although the undertaking may be challenging, the potential benefits are substantial, including enhanced group unity, increased motivation, and a significant advancement in overall productivity.

The "Empathy Ripple Effect" phenomenon entails a sustained dedication characterized by many challenges and moments of significant progress. However, this transformative journey is of great value since it has the potential to impact individual interactions and reshape the nature of military leadership.

As the propagation of empathy traverses all echelons of leadership, extending from individual troops to cohesive teams, and further encompassing entire military organizations, it constructs a compelling narrative that exemplifies the optimal state of the military—marked by humanity, compassion, and remarkable efficacy. As we progress, it is imperative that we not only engage in the examination of this phenomenon but also actively engage in its progression. Allow the propagation of the ripple effect and let us bear witness to the tremendous transformations that empathy has the potential to initiate.

CHAPTER 8

BEYOND RANK: BUILDING TRUST THROUGH EMPATHY

Within military settings, the concept of rank serves as an indisputable factor in establishing power, a formalization of accountability, and a fundamental framework for organizational structure. It serves as the structural framework on which the establishment of military discipline, organization, and ranking is built. Nevertheless, it is vital to comprehend that hierarchy alone is an inadequate tool for fostering trust, which is the fundamental basis for the formation of effective teams. Trust can be considered as a phenomenon that arises from genuine interpersonal relationships, surpassing the structured nature of military hierarchies. The development of empathy is essential for individuals to thrive, as it requires a more complex and compassionate quality.

Empathy functions as a valuable complement to the otherwise rigid hierarchical structure. This statement highlights the presence of human qualities throughout every level of the military hierarchy. Regardless of their position, each person is a multifaceted combination of emotions, goals, anxieties, and hopes. A leader possessing empathic intelligence surpasses the constrained scope of hierarchical power. A leader of this nature exemplifies a dualistic function, encompassing both the responsibilities of a commanding officer and the position of a mentor. This individual serves as an authoritative presence while also fostering a collaborative environment as a team member. The leader strives to understand the diverse viewpoints within their team, empathize with their difficulties, acknowledge their strengths, and offer support for their individual obstacles.

Take, for example, Colonel Elena Rodriguez, who took charge of a unit that had a notoriously underwhelming track record and diminishing morale. Instead of implementing a harsh and oppressive system, Colonel

Rodriguez introduced a program called "Leadership Circles." This initiative provided a platform for individuals of different ranks to engage in open discussions regarding operational and personal issues, as well as explore alternative solutions. The environment, characterized by its unique approach of promoting equal communication among individuals of different hierarchical positions, provided team members with a feeling of empowerment and affirmation. Furthermore, this occurrence brought about a significant change in their perspective of Rodriguez, transitioning him from an inscrutable figure of power to a compassionate leader dedicated to collaborative resolution of issues and the welfare of the group. Following the aforementioned events, the battalion witnessed a notable increase in operational efficiency, accompanied by a significant strengthening of trust within the team.

The expression of empathy serves as a means via which trust is built. When military personnel experience genuine appreciation and understanding that goes beyond their assigned positions or levels, it leads to an increased inclination to place trust in others. Individuals tend to be more receptive to the instruction of a leader who demonstrates understanding, more inclined to trust a commander who exemplifies empathy, and more internally motivated to achieve in their responsibilities for a leader who recognizes their uniqueness.

Establishing an empathetic culture inside the military paradigm is a complex undertaking. It necessitates a delicate balance between upholding hierarchical power structures and fostering a setting that promotes emotional openness, between exercising control and encouraging inclusive discourse, and between giving directions and seeking valuable input.
Nevertheless, once well maneuvered, the outcome is a type of confidence that surpasses the boundaries imposed by

hierarchical positions within the armed forces. It fosters a powerful combination of steadfast allegiance, integrated solidarity, and a mutually beneficial perception of shared objectives and intentions. The establishment of trust not only fosters a strong sense of unity among the team, but also has the potential to fundamentally reshape the fundamental nature of military leadership.

As the investigation into the complex domain of empathetic military leadership progresses, it becomes increasingly apparent that the interplay between empathy and trust holds significant transformational capabilities. It possesses the capability to not only enhance operational efficiency but also initiate a transformative change in the principles that govern military leadership. Let us persist in exploring this rich domain and see the transforming combination of empathy and trust—a fusion that holds the capacity to cultivate a type of military leadership that is both deeply attuned to emotions and highly skilled in strategic decision-making.

CHAPTER 9

EMPATHY IN CRISIS: MANAGING STRESS AND TRAUMA

A crisis's unfiltered and unrelenting nature exposes the essential elements of leadership. As mentioned above, the phenomenon functions as a discerning instrument, exposing both the capabilities and susceptibilities of those in positions of power. As a leader, individuals face many challenges that progressively increase in complexity, growing more difficult in their nature.

The scope of responsibility encompasses a wide range of tasks, including managing challenging weather conditions, optimizing the allocation and usage of resources, and making tough decisions that might be emotionally challenging. Every decision made and strategy followed bears the responsibility of determining the entire team's outcome.

However, the core of crisis leadership extends beyond mere tactical choices or the maintenance of stability. The genuine assessment is in one's capacity to effectively manage the diverse range of human emotions that arise during challenging circumstances. This pertains to the comprehension and resolution of emotions such as dread, confusion, and hopelessness, which frequently remain concealed but are intensely brewing beneath the exterior, eagerly anticipating a leader's authentic recognition.

During the present period, characterized by unpredictability and disruption, leadership that demonstrates empathy emerges as a comforting and therapeutic influence. Leaders who exemplify empathy distinguish themselves not only as individuals in positions of authority or as individuals responsible for making decisions but also as individuals who possess a deep understanding and sensitivity towards the emotional well-being of their teams.

A leader of this kind does not disregard the potential impact of emotional upheaval that may influence the team. In contrast, individuals acknowledge these emotional states, actively listen attentively, and respond with suitable and prompt measures. This authentic recognition and subsequent reaction establish the basis for trust, a fundamental element for achieving success in any undertaking.

Leaders play a pivotal role in validating individuals by building an emotional connection. The conveyed message is of great significance, as it emphasizes the authenticity, genuineness, and utmost importance of every team member's emotions and experiences. This phenomenon serves as evidence of a shared sense of community, highlighting the notion that, when confronted with obstacles, individuals are joined in a cohesive manner, collectively embarking on the same path.

This association enhances leaders' understanding, enabling them to support their teams effectively. Organizations that adopt and incorporate this comprehension are strategically positioned to gain a competitive edge. These individuals exhibit a distinct ability to conduct a more comprehensive assessment of the emotional state of their constituents, hence prioritizing the welfare of the individuals involved.

Given this comprehension, the methodology undergoes a transformation. The focus has shifted away from inflexible strategies. However, it highlights the importance of modifying approaches to address and alleviate stress while also considering the varied emotional requirements of every individual involved. This proactive approach seeks to establish stability in advance, prior to the occurrence of a storm.

Nevertheless, the scope of responsibility for these compassionate leaders extends beyond basic problem-solving. They are not merely leading their squad out of the state of chaos. The organization's main goal is to equip its team members with the necessary resources and knowledge to effectively traverse challenging circumstances, ensuring that each individual emerges from these experiences unharmed and develops increased strength and resilience.

Leaders often face difficulties in striking a careful balance between empathy and power. Achieving an optimal equilibrium is of utmost importance. An abundance of empathy has the potential to blur the distinct boundary between a leader and their team. The lack of clear distinction between roles and responsibilities could result in a progressive decline of the leader's influence, jeopardizing their ability to remain unbiased and render impartial judgments.

Conversely, a dearth of empathy might provide an equally challenging issue. The phenomenon has the potential to intensify the emotional disconnect between the leader and their team, resulting in a climate characterized by detachment and disillusionment. The presence of a leader who exhibits a lack of concern or detachment has the potential to undermine trust and diminish morale among members of the organization.

Hence, the fundamental nature of empathic leadership does not involve excessively leaning towards any certain way. The attainment of a delicate equilibrium is required. Achieving equilibrium in this context entails a harmonious interaction between cultivating authentic relationships and imposing authoritative control. The ability to comprehend alternative viewpoints while also possessing the determination to enact essential actions is crucial.

Despite the various difficulties, it is obvious that there are significant benefits associated with the incorporation of empathic leadership into the field of crisis management. Fundamentally, this particular leadership approach possesses the capacity to shape a team that not only demonstrates resilience, but also leverages a crisis as an opportunity for advancement and development. A team that is formed under the leadership of empathy is not only enduring the challenges it faces, but also acquiring the ability to effectively utilize them.

One notable advantage is the augmentation of trust. During times of crisis, characterized by significant uncertainty, trust plays a fundamental role in providing a solid foundation for the team. It serves as the cohesive force that fosters a sense of unity and prevents any individual from experiencing a sense of detachment or seclusion.

Another significant result is the promotion of efficient communication. A leader who possesses empathy fosters a conducive atmosphere wherein team members experience a sense of being acknowledged and esteemed. The importance of open communication lines is particularly pronounced when dealing with complex situations during a crisis.

Furthermore, the promotion of cooperation is a result that must not be disregarded. Even in the most difficult circumstances, a team that is guided by empathy demonstrates enhanced collaboration, as they effectively combine their collective resources and knowledge.

Empathic leadership, fundamentally, imbues situations that may occasionally appear devoid of humanity with a deep feeling of compassion and understanding. The incorporation of emotional intelligence is seamlessly integrated into the complex framework of crisis management. As we navigate the complex landscape of military operations, the significance of empathy becomes readily apparent. The process of effective leadership involves more than simply issuing directives from a hierarchical position. It necessitates a comprehensive comprehension of the human factor that is intricately interwoven within each strategic approach and decision-making process.

In the present situation, empathy is not a gratuitous luxury, but rather an essential requirement. It serves as a mediator, bridging the divide between authoritative instructions and genuine empathy, as well as between the overarching mission goals and the individuals entrusted with their attainment. Similar to how a compass is deemed essential for a sailor navigating tumultuous waters, empathy serves as a guiding force for leaders under the turbulent circumstances of a crisis.

CHAPTER 10

EMPATHY VOID: A WRITER'S LIVED EXPERIENCE

EMPATHY HAS NO RANK

In 2021, after nearly two decades in the military, I confronted challenges that reshaped my understanding of leadership and humanity. It's said, "You don't know what you don't know," and I realized that once enlightened, we must decide to evolve or stagnate. Throughout my military career, from combat to providing mental health care in conflict zones, I observed that our institution frequently learns through tough experiences. From these rigorous lessons, we pivot and strive for better outcomes.

This personal evolution became glaringly apparent in my leadership style, where I grappled with my understanding of empathy. While I perceived my unit as compassionate, my view on empathy's significance was rather muted. On the other hand, my team held empathy in high regard, even if it wasn't always expressed overtly. This disparity made me reflect on the origins of my limited empathy.

Empathy, I've come to realize, isn't black and white. It operates on a spectrum. My Achilles heel was a lack of patience for personal matters, while I was more considerate about professional challenges. By contrast, some leaders I've encountered seem broadly unempathetic, dialing down their emotional responses.

Rooted in my challenging upbringing, my diminished empathy served as a protective shield. Keeping emotions at arm's length felt safer. This emotional distance inadvertently stunted my connections with family, colleagues, and friends. It hampered my ability to understand diverse perspectives, curbing adaptability, a trait crucial for effective leadership.

This disconnect often led me to self-isolation. I dulled my emotional intelligence by doing so, struggling to resonate with others' feelings and experiences. A creeping belief began to set in: I was the sole protagonist in my narrative, and others' emotions were less significant. This sense of isolation and self-centeredness further widened the gap between me and the world around me.

EMPATHY HAS NO RANK

Without the compass of empathy, communication became a labyrinth. True communication requires an understanding of the speaker's emotions, the context, and the listener's state of mind. My inability to tune into these nuances often resulted in misunderstandings, inadvertently sowing discord and misperceptions, which undermined my professional relationships.

In reflection, 2021 taught me the invaluable lesson of the power and necessity of empathy, not just as a leader but as a human being.

In my journey as a military leader, I've come to realize that genuine connections are built on more than just authority or rank; they hinge on our ability to truly connect with others. At the heart of this connection lies empathy, a cornerstone of Emotional Intelligence, which I once overlooked in my drive for professional success. Candidly, my career climbs were often self-centered. But upon introspection, I uncovered four profound reasons for my blind spot around empathy, an insight that has reshaped my leadership approach.

1. **I'm a fixer**
   I've carried the insignia of a "fixer" with pride throughout my life and career. Hand me a problem, and my mind immediately leaps into action, tirelessly churning through potential solutions, strategies, and pathways to resolution. This ability has always been my greatest asset, distinguishing me in numerous situations. I've come to realize, however, that while the fixer mentality is a valuable asset, it can also be a double-edged weapon, particularly in leadership positions.

   I still have a recent memory of an incident. Almost as if my mind were hardwired to skip to the finish line. When confronted with obstacles, I rarely linger in the problem space. Instead, I transition swiftly to identifying actionable measures to resolve the problem at hand. This rapid troubleshooting style occasionally became my Achilles' heel, especially when managing and working with coworkers.

There was an incident that is still fresh in my mind. A distressed member of my team approached me for guidance. As they began to describe their predicament, my mind, true to form, was already three steps ahead, formulating solutions, anticipating potential obstacles, and mentally preparing a course of action. I was prepared with my proposed solution by the time they completed their narrative. However, their demeanor caused me to hesitate. They appeared more burdened than before, as if my rapid resolution had exacerbated their situation rather than alleviated it.

This interaction was a pivotal moment in my life. I recognized that my efficient fixer mentality frequently prevented me from truly listening. I used to think that whenever somebody approached me having a problem, they were probably looking for a solution. But for the majority of the time, they preferred someone who would actually pay listen, comprehend their situation, and provide support.

In addition, in my haste to provide solutions, I inadvertently deprived individuals of their autonomy. Instead of empowering them to take responsibility for their issues and encouraging them to consider potential solutions, I was inadvertently increasing their reliance on me. This was detrimental to their development and my leadership role.

I learned over time the significance of restraint and the value of attentive listening. When given the opportunity to express their concerns and work through their emotions, a great number of individuals often arrive at a solution on their own. They are seeking validation, comprehension, and sometimes just a sounding board from their leader, not necessarily a resolution.

I began to ask individuals open-ended questions in an effort to encourage them to reflect on their challenges and consider potential solutions after I slowed down my instinctive desire to solve problems. This strategy not only boosted their confidence, but also ensured that they retained responsibility and ownership of the issue. It was a profound realization that sometimes the best way to assist someone is to guide them in discovering their own solutions rather than providing them with your own.

The transition from problem solver to empathic listener has been both challenging and enlightening. While problem-solving will always be a part of my DNA, I've come to comprehend the nuances of leadership and the significance of truly listening. Sometimes, leadership involves guiding individuals to discover their own solutions, empowering them, and cultivating an atmosphere of trust and mutual respect. As I continue in my leadership role, I endeavor to strike a balance between my fixer instincts and the invaluable skill of empathetic listening, constantly reminding myself that solutions are essential, but so is the process of achieving them.

2. **All about the mission**
   As a mental health officer and flight commander at a military mental health facility, I have consistently been imbued with a deep sense of duty and accountability. The paramount concern of the mission's gravity and the preservation of service personnel' mental well-being became the central focal point, frequently eclipsing individual intricacies and feelings. I had the belief that maintaining a laser-like focus on the purpose was a fundamental component of my leadership approach. Nevertheless, as time has passed, I have developed a comprehension that prioritizing the purpose is of utmost importance; however, disregarding the individual wants and concerns of my subordinates might have adverse effects on productivity.

Within the context of the military, the attribute of being mission-driven is frequently commended and held in high regard. The aforementioned attributes of dedication, discipline, and an unshakeable commitment serve as symbolic representations of one's allegiance to the objectives of our nation. As the individual in a position of leadership inside a mental health clinic, this particular attribute appeared to be of heightened significance. On a daily basis, I engaged with individuals who had diverse obstacles, and I held the belief that promptly assisting them in resolving their issues to regain focus on the purpose was the most effective strategy. However, due to my fervor in resolving the issue, I frequently overlooked the individual involved in it.

One vivid example is etched in my recollection. An somebody at a lower position, displaying clear signs of discomfort, contacted me to express a concern. Mentally, I had already begun formulating strategies to address the problem, aiming to steer their focus back towards our overarching purpose. I provided several answers, tactics, and personal tales pertaining to analogous circumstances, with the intention of facilitating their prompt restoration to an ideal state of performance. Nevertheless, with the culmination of the discourse, I discerned a significant disparity. Rather than experiencing a sense of being listened to and comprehended, the individuals appeared to be increasingly isolated, displaying visible signs of diminished confidence in the mission and myself as their leader.

Upon engaging in moments of introspection, I came to the realization of my error. Inadvertently, my intense dedication to the purpose resulted in the unintentional disregard for the individual's personal experience. Due to my impulsive approach in seeking a resolution, I neglected to sincerely engage in active listening, comprehend their emotions, and demonstrate empathy towards their viewpoint. The individuals in question were not merely in search of a temporary solution, but rather sought validation, comprehension, and the guarantee that their leader held a genuine concern for their overall well.

EMPATHY HAS NO RANK

Within the military, an often used phrase is "Mission First, People Always." Although I consistently comprehended the initial segment, the profound significance of the later frequently evaded my understanding. The execution of a mission, regardless of its level of importance, is carried out by individuals. These individuals, characterized by their distinct experiences, emotions, and challenges, require more than mere instructions. Individuals strive to attain comprehension, affirmation, and authentic interpersonal bonds.

In the realm of mental health, leaders who prioritize their objective above all else may occasionally overlook the individual experiences and personal growth of their subordinates. The significance lies not only in achieving the desired outcome, but also in fostering a sense of inclusivity, recognition, and true commitment among all individuals involved in the endeavor.

Throughout my experience as a flight commander, I have acquired an understanding of the need of incorporating pauses, actively listening, and providing individuals with the opportunity to reflect about and articulate their emotions. The process involves not merely hastening through a situation, but rather comprehending it thoroughly, acknowledging the emotions experienced by the individual, and thereafter working together to build a collective plan for moving forward. This strategy not only cultivates trust and a sense of camaraderie, but also guarantees that the mission is backed by individuals who experience acknowledgment, active listening, and appreciation.

In summary, effective leadership, particularly within the domains of the military, necessitates a nuanced equilibrium between maintaining a strong focus on objectives and demonstrating authentic empathy. The mission statement serves as a guiding principle, although it is the individuals involved, their dedication, confidence, and welfare, that genuinely propel its progress. In the course of my ongoing service, I consistently bear in mind the knowledge acquired, consistently reinforcing the notion that although the mission holds paramount importance, it is ultimately the individuals involved who hold the utmost significance. In my capacity as a leader, I bear the obligation not just towards the overarching objectives, but also towards each individual who has placed their trust in me for their welfare and personal development.

3. **I was defensive**

    Reflecting on my years of military service as an officer, a recurring pattern emerges: my heightened sense of defensiveness. This characteristic, which initially appeared to be a protective mechanism, became a significant barrier to establishing genuine connections with my subordinates and to expressing genuine empathy.

As the leader of a mission, surrounded by responsibilities and performance pressure, I subconsciously erected a defensive wall. I believed that obstacles impeded advancement. In my mind, I was laboring tirelessly to ensure the success of our mission. The notion of stopping to address individual concerns felt like an unwarranted detour, consuming precious time and resources. My first reaction? A defensive stance. A natural, almost reflexive urge to protect oneself from potential threats, criticisms, or impediments. My default perception was that every concern was an enemy of the mission.

Being defensive is a challenge since it is driven by the need to protect oneself. Although it gives the appearance of security, it restricts our viewpoint. I regarded challenges and criticisms as direct confrontations rather than opportunities for growth and comprehension. In doing so, I was unable to identify the underlying emotions, concerns, or requirements that initially prompted these challenges.

Unfortunately, this defensive perspective impeded my capacity for empathy. Empathy requires openness, vulnerability, and the capacity to put oneself in another's circumstances. Empathy fosters genuine understanding and connection; however, my defensiveness prevented me from seeing beyond my own perspective.

A painful memory that underscores the impact of my defensiveness was a meeting that took place in 2021. A co-worker took me aside after perceiving the rising tension and hostile environment I was inadvertently creating. During the meeting, I was warned against adopting such a confrontational stance. This fleeting interruption in time left an indelible impression on my mind.

In lieu of adopting my usual defensive posture, I chose to adopt a neutral, almost passive stance in response to the presented problem. I did not attempt to defend our mission or my position. This transition in approach brought about a remarkable transformation. By withdrawing, I made room for others to advance. Surprisingly, people rallied behind the mission and even defended it when I didn't.

This experience illuminated profound insights. The mere fact that someone poses a problem or raises a concern does not necessarily imply that they oppose the mission or objective. Frequently, these obstacles are the result of genuine concerns, shared objectives, or a desire to improve the mission's success.

This realization prompted me to ponder the numerous instances in which my defensiveness may have suppressed valuable feedback or prevented a subordinate from sharing a brilliant insight. How often had I inadvertently erected a barrier to comprehension because I was too armored?

Leadership requires more than simply navigating a ship through tranquil waters. It involves navigating through disasters, comprehending the crew's concerns, and ensuring that everyone feels seen, heard, and valued. While defensiveness may provide a temporary shield, empathy is what truly connects a leader to his or her team, fostering trust, understanding, and a shared sense of purpose.

I carry the lessons from that pivotal meeting with me as I proceed forward. I am reminded of the power of vulnerability, the importance of putting aside defensiveness in order to genuinely listen, and the extraordinary things that can occur when one allows others to contribute. While the process of shedding my defensive nature is ongoing, I am committed to cultivating an atmosphere of understanding, empathy, and collective development.

4. **I spoke more than I listened**
Amidst the clamor of requests and the burdensome idea of the military, I've understood that I talk more than I tune in. This mindfulness didn't foster for the time being, but instead through a progression of occasions that incited me to consider my correspondence style and its effect on my subordinates.

There are numerous factors why I have this tendency. Most importantly, having a sense of authority and duty as an officer in the armed forces is a given. This has unintentionally led me to develop the belief that my voice, thoughts, and choices are crucial over time. Inadvertently, I have frequently regarded my perspective as the most essential and as the one that should dominate conversations.

In addition, the military environment is based on discipline, hierarchy, and swift decision making. In critical situations, lengthy discussions are not always possible; orders must be issued swiftly and carried out immediately. This has further ingrained in me the habit of speaking with confidence and authority. Unfortunately, there are times when the line between these crucial moments and everyday interactions becomes hazy.

Nevertheless, my tendency to speak more than listen originates from a profound fear of exposure. To listen, to genuinely listen, one must be vulnerable. It necessitates a readiness to change, a willingness to listen to alternative viewpoints, and the courage to admit one could be wrong. And on rare occasions, admitting mistakes might seem like a show of weakness for someone in my position of responsibility.

My youthful subordinate was involved in an incident that vividly illustrates the negative implications of my communication style. She approached me with the intent of discussing a situation she believed I had mishandled. It was evident from her hesitant demeanor and careful word selection that the matter was of great significance to her.

However, rather than allowing her the space and time to articulate her thoughts and concerns, I immediately defended myself. I never paused to truly comprehend her perspective, obscuring her voice with explanations and justifications of my own. My impatience and inability to simply listen hindered my ability to develop empathy.

This interaction's aftermath was a clear indication of my inability to communicate. Not only did my relationship with this particular subordinate become fraught, but word of the incident spread throughout the ranks, fostering mistrust and trepidation. I realized that by not actively listening, not only had I disregarded her emotions, but I had also inadvertently conveyed to all my subordinates that their voices did not matter.

In essence, my tendency to communicate more than I listen compromised the very foundation of leadership - trust. A leader who does not listen has no chance of inspiring, motivating, or connecting with his or her team. I risked alienating those who looked to me for guidance and support by prioritizing my opinion over theirs.

In retrospect, my position necessitates not only respect and authority, but also understanding and compassion. Despite its structured exterior, the military is composed of individuals with emotions, concerns, and requirements. In this circumstance, listening involves hearing words as well as understanding the intentions and motives underlying them.

I've got the chance to learn quite a bit about myself on this challenging journey. Despite the fact that the road to improving my listening skills is lengthy and plain, it is still uncertain whether or not to expend the necessary effort. As Stephen R. Covey said, "the majority of individuals don't pay attention with a desire to comprehend what is being said; they pay attention with the objective to respond." Being a part of the first group, which constantly seeks to understand before striving to be understood, is my goal.

CHAPTER 11

GET ACTIVE: EMPATHY SKILLS FOR LEADERS

Empathy Guarantees Good Communication

Empathy is a fundamental element that plays a crucial role in ensuring the efficacy of interpersonal communication, extending beyond being merely a popular term or catchphrase. Leaders who demonstrate a commitment to empathy actively engage in comprehending and appreciating their subordinates' viewpoints. Despite potential disagreements, individuals accept differing opinions, refrain from passing judgment, and consistently consider the underlying emotions and experiences that shape these perspectives.

This attribute facilitates comprehension and establishes a bedrock of confidence among team members. By establishing a conducive atmosphere wherein every individual is esteemed and given a platform for expression, leaders who possess empathy inherently facilitate the development of a work environment characterized by collaboration and unity.

In addition, persons who exhibit empathy demonstrate an increased level of sensitivity towards nonverbal signs. Individuals possess the ability to perceive and interpret nuanced cues, such as facial expressions or fluctuations in vocal intonation. This inherent comprehension enables individuals to assess the emotions and requirements of their team members with more precision, so enabling the provision of appropriate assistance at the appropriate moment.

Empathy Helps Resolve Conflicts

According to Diana Francis, it can be observed that in circumstances when change is not only unavoidable but also preferable, conflict becomes an unavoidable occurrence. This profound assertion holds significant resonance within the context of enterprises and organizations, whereby divergent viewpoints regarding projects or contracts are an inherent and commonplace phenomenon.

In such situations, leaders who demonstrate empathy exhibit notable qualities. Demonstrating a heightened awareness of their environment, individuals exhibit an almost prophetic aptitude in discerning forthcoming disputes within their professional teams. This ability to anticipate future events allows individuals to respond promptly, addressing problems at an early stage to prevent their escalation. Understanding the nuances of human feelings and actions is just as important as taking an aggressive strategy.

The leaders in question are highly respected by their fellow workers, who regularly show admiration for their judgment and approach. By possessing a profound understanding of the dynamics inside their team, individuals are able to anticipate the potential reactions of employees in certain situations. The possession of such analytical qualities enables individuals to engage in diplomatic approaches, so facilitating the management of conflicts through the use of understanding and sensitivity.

Empathy allows you to have an overview
Empathetic leaders demonstrate a distinctive combination of steadfast dedication to the organization's purpose and a deep comprehension of their employees' viewpoints and feelings. The individual's capacity to maintain steadfastness in their convictions, while also demonstrating sensitivity towards the perspectives and emotions of their colleagues, distinguishes them from others.

A comprehensive study, involving more than 15,000 leaders from diverse corners of the globe, has underscored empathy as the primary catalyst for employee performance. However, what is the underlying reason for the immense potency of empathy? It allows leaders to align their long-term aims with the immediate goals they need to achieve. When faced with initiatives that have the potential to become complex and confusing, these leaders have exceptional skills in simplifying and clarifying, so ensuring clarity throughout the process.

Furthermore, these proficient leaders exhibit a heightened sense of self-awareness. The individuals acknowledge the cascading impact of their emotional states on the entirety of the company. The emotional resonance described here serves as a powerful motivator, acting as a catalyst that significantly contributes to the overall success of the firm.

How Leaders Can Be Empathetic

Consider the importance of being empathetic at work. Although empathy has long been acknowledged as a valuable trait in the business domain, it is concerning to observe the number of leaders who have not fully comprehended its profound importance or how to authentically manifest it inside the workplace. There is a common misconception among individuals that emotional expression is synonymous with vulnerability or a lack of strength. However, genuine emotional involvement has the potential to foster increased trust and rapport among team members.

The use of empathy enables leaders to effectively perceive and comprehend the difficulties and requirements of their team members. Consider, for example, an employee who experiences a delay in their work attendance as a result of a family emergency. Rather than exhibiting a reflexive and negative reaction centered around the failure to meet a deadline, a leader who demonstrates empathy would place importance on the employee's welfare, providing comprehension and assistance. These actions significantly impact cultivating a work atmosphere that promotes support and collaboration.

A common mistake observed among managers is their tendency to prioritize outcomes over the process. This perspective has the unintended consequence of reducing the perceived worth of an employee's commitment and diligent efforts. Through the incorporation of empathy, a leader gains enhanced capabilities to identify the underlying factors contributing to declines in performance. Numerous elements, including personal challenges, health issues, financial pressures, and learning difficulties, can influence an employee's productivity.

Leaders may need help effectively inspiring and guiding their employees if they take the time to contemplate the root reasons for their challenges and provide support. Although highly important, authentic empathy necessitates the exercise of patience and a committed endeavor to comprehend a wide range of viewpoints and emotions. In order to enhance one's leadership skills and cultivate a greater sense of empathy towards one's team members, it is advisable to explore the following insights and recommendations.

1: Practice Active Listening
In a military environment, it's critical to provide team members with the regard and consideration they deserve when they visit you. Due to the numerous duties that come along with a military commander, such as overseeing employees, distributing resources, and meeting stringent deadlines, it is normal to feel overburdened. It is crucial to create a situation free of distractions to understand the essence of a service member's apprehension completely. Use preventative measures like removing your Common Access Card (CAC) from your computer, moving away from your workstation, and making sure there are no physical barriers in the way of the individual you are interacting with. One can communicate to their subordinates that they are engaged and carefully absorbing information by making and maintaining regular eye contact and using non-verbal signs like nodding. The words being communicated may be understood, but is the underlying feeling being internalized? It may be beneficial to engage in the practice of pausing, reflecting, and making sure that the message's main points are well understood.

Active listening is not only a showy behavior but a vital skill that sets a leader apart from a manager. Genuine interest in team members' thoughts involves more than just listening; it also involves understanding and appreciating their perspectives and concerns. In the framework of armed forces activities, where the growth of collaboration and confidence is of the highest significance, such acts assist in the growth of relationships among individuals.

The benefits of listening to what is being expressed extend beyond the immediate environment as well. The importance of this element in boosting a company's performance cannot be overstated. The foundation for the growth of mutual trust is laid by creating a cultural environment that values the practice of active listening. This culture not only enhances corporate culture. This approach encourages productivity improvement and offers resources for successfully handling and resolving conflicts. Precision and coordination are extremely important in military circumstances because they have the ability to produce significant results.

2: Do Not Interrupt
An essential element of effective empathetic leadership involves the practice of abstaining from interrupting others. In order to properly embody this idea, it is imperative to actively participate in the dialogue by utilizing all sensory faculties, so ensuring complete presence during the interaction. Prior to constructing a reply or succumbing to potential diversions, such as engaging with one's mobile device, it is advisable to fully engage in the ongoing conversation. Engaging in the act of shuffling papers or exhibiting a lack of focus throughout the process of someone presenting their perspective can potentially communicate a sense of disinterest or impatience.

It is not uncommon for individuals, particularly in fast-paced workplaces, to experience impatience and seek to accelerate the speed of discourse. Nevertheless, this can unintentionally lead to the speaker experiencing a sense of diminished worth. When faced with a situation when there are other urgent chores or an impending meeting, it is considered more courteous to express the limitations or constraints that prevent immediate action. Recognize the significance of the discourse, convey remorse, and offer apologies for the inability to allocate the requisite attention at present. By adopting this approach, individuals can effectively establish and uphold channels of communication, while concurrently demonstrating a commitment to treating others with courtesy and understanding.

3: Manage Your Body Language
Non-verbal cues possess a remarkable capacity to convey meaning that surpasses the impact of verbal communication. When interacting with someone, it is imperative to maintain awareness of one's nonverbal communication cues. The importance of displaying politeness extends beyond mere appearances, as it encompasses the sincere expression of one's involvement and enthusiasm towards the conveyed message. Please pause for a moment to consider how you would want someone to approach you when you are sharing your ideas. How might experiencing someone's posture, facial expressions, and hand gestures help one feel as like they are actively being heard and valued?

The subtleties of nonverbal communication, specifically body language, possess significant predictive value in discerning an individual's emotional condition or degree of engagement. Indicators of disengagement or boredom have the potential to swiftly manifest themselves, even in the most inconspicuous forms of nonverbal communication. In light of the increasing prevalence of remote or hybrid work arrangements in various organizations, the need of comprehending these indications is further underscored. In both virtual and in-person settings, it is feasible to perceive indications of dejection, disconnection, or frustration in a colleague only through their physical manifestations.

Developing proficiency in the realm of nonverbal communication is crucial for fostering empathic leadership. Nonverbal cues, like as gestures and postures, possess the capacity to convey significant information regarding an individual's level of engagement within a conversation. In addition to nonverbal cues such as bodily gestures, vocal tone and modulation are also significant factors in the process of communication. The vocal expression of a leader has the potential to convey sentiments of warmth, understanding, and encouragement, or conversely, may unintentionally manifest indications of frustration and disinterest.

In order to effectively inspire and motivate a team, it is imperative for a leader to possess sympathetic qualities and demonstrate a high level of engagement. This entails being fully present and employing both verbal and non-verbal forms of communication to convey support, encouragement, and understanding. The following are a selection of refined tactics that can be employed to augment non-verbal communication skills in the context of empathic leadership:

Maintain an open posture by refraining from crossing your arms. An open attitude is characterized by its inviting nature and serves as an indicator of receptiveness.

Maintaining consistent eye contact is crucial during interpersonal communication, particularly when an individual is speaking. This rudimentary action demonstrates one's active engagement in the act of listening and the recognition of the significance of the information being shared.

1: Vocal modulation is an essential aspect of effective communication, characterized by the ability to articulate words clearly and keep a composed and consistent tone throughout speech. This demonstrates a sense of self-assurance and poise.

2: The Significance of Authentic Smiles: The potency of a grin lies in its authenticity. It is advisable to ensure that one's smiles are timely and genuine, effectively aligning with the present discourse.

3: Maintaining a Relaxed Body Language: It is advisable to refrain from exhibiting signs of tension or rigidity. A posture that is characterized by a lack of rigidity and tension conveys a sense of ease and receptiveness in the context of a conversation.

By incorporating these methods into your interpersonal exchanges, you will progress towards embodying empathetic leadership, cultivating a culture characterized by trust, comprehension, and reciprocal regard.

4: Let go of Prejudice
The adoption of an open-minded perspective is essential for cultivating a flourishing and inclusive work environment. This involves the act of refraining from adopting inflexible attitudes or forming premature assessments. In a workplace characterized by diversity, it is inevitable that one may face a multitude of perspectives, some of which may deviate considerably from one's own. This guide provides strategies for effectively navigating such situations with tact and comprehension.

Cultivate a Receptive Attitude:: Try to engage in discussions without preexisting assumptions. Each connection presents a potential for personal development and acquisition of knowledge. By approaching a conversation without preconceived biases, individuals provide opportunities for the emergence of novel ideas and unique viewpoints.

Cherish Diversity of Thought: It is important to recognize that diversity encompasses more than just demographic differences but also the wide range of perspectives and ideas that individuals bring. While it is inherent for individuals to be drawn toward others with similar beliefs, there is significant merit in engaging with individuals with contrasting perspectives. They can introduce novel approaches, so expanding our perspectives.

Exercise Tolerance: This concept is necessary to demonstrate respect and patience towards divergent perspectives. The concept of tolerance entails neither agreement nor endorsement but rather encompasses the recognition and comprehension of alternative perspectives distinct from one's own.

Engage Deeply: In order to fully comprehend the messages being conveyed by one's team members, it is advisable to engage in active listening techniques. Kindly provide further information, seek further clarification, and request specific instances to enhance understanding. This demonstrates a genuine interest on your part and facilitates a more comprehensive comprehension of the context and intricacies of the information being conveyed.

Resist Rushed Judgments: In order to cultivate a compassionate leadership style, it is crucial to acknowledge the significance of engaging in attentive and patient listening, thereby refraining from hastily forming judgments. By abstaining from making hasty judgments, one creates room for a thorough comprehension. The act of active listening involves more than simply waiting for an opportunity to speak; rather, it entails fully engaging with and embracing the narrative of the interlocutor.

Empathetic leadership is fundamentally rooted in the principles of comprehension and interpersonal bonding. By placing genuine importance on and deeply assimilating the ideas and perspectives contributed by your team members, you cultivate a setting characterized by trust, cooperation, and reciprocal regard.

5: This of "we" instead of "me"
Fostering a team-centric leadership style can have a significant impact

on the morale and productivity of your employees. Here is a comprehensive guide to cultivating this perspective:

Adopt a Collective Mindset: Begin by reframing your decision-making process in terms of "we" as opposed to "I." When strategizing or planning, constantly contemplate on what's optimal for the entire group. Consider queries such as "How will this benefit the team?" and "How might the team respond to this shift?"

Promote Inclusivity in Decision-making: True empathy in leadership extends beyond comprehension; it entails valuing and including the voices of your team in decision-making, particularly when such decisions directly affect them. Participate in brainstorming sessions with them, elicit their input, and make them feel more like stakeholders than mere executors.

Differentiate between 'Boss' and 'Leader': A 'boss' typically dictates, monitors, and regulates, frequently leading from a position of authority as opposed to influence. A 'leader,' on the other hand, motivates, instructs, and encourages teamwork. The latter strategy tends to generate greater team commitment and engagement.

Overcome Traditional Barriers: It is crucial to recognize that certain organizational structures and cultures may inherently favor the 'master' mentality. For example, reluctance to implement remote work may result from a desire for control. Recognize these traditional obstacles and make proactive efforts to overcome them.

Encourage Autonomy and Growth: One of the negative effects of a "boss" mentality is the suppression of innovation and individual development. A relaxed, top-down approach can allow employees to fully utilize their skills and expertise. In contrast, an empathic leader promotes autonomy, enabling employees to realize their maximum potential and contribute in a more holistic manner.

Foster a Positive Work Environment: Beyond tasks and projects, a workplace's overall atmosphere significantly impacts productivity and happiness. A more positive and productive atmosphere is likely to encourage open communication, respect diverse opinions, and value every contribution, regardless of hierarchy.

In essence, shifting from a "boss" mentality to a "leader" mentality involves a transformation in approach, perspective, and interaction that prioritizes the group over the individual. This development results in a more harmonious, productive, and inventive workplace.

6: Don't be afraid of Mistakes

The essence of human nature entails an inherent fallibility and susceptibility to committing errors. It is necessary to promote a collaborative environment that admits mistakes, takes part in group discussion, and successfully executes initiatives.

By openly acknowledging an error in the presence of others, you establish a significant precedent. The demonstration of transparency has the potential to serve as a source of inspiration for individuals in one's vicinity, so encouraging them to embrace vulnerability and acknowledge their personal limitations. It cultivates a societal environment characterized by principles of integrity and emotional openness.

Additionally, it is important to take aggressive steps to address and correct faults rather than just admitting them. It is crucial to promote an organizational spirit that accepts mistakes, participates in collaborative brainstorming, and implements ideas successfully. This method not only effectively tackles the immediate issue at hand, but also makes a valuable contribution to the overall growth and development.

7: Get Training in Business Leadership

Individuals do not possess inherent knowledge of all subjects upon birth, and this notion is particularly applicable within the domains of business and leadership. Engaging in corporate leadership training is a crucial step for individuals aspiring to cultivate sympathetic leadership qualities. This course equips individuals with the fundamental principles and resources required to foster comprehension, benevolence, and authentic empathy for the individuals under their guidance.

Flourishing teams that develop into self-sufficient entities frequently exhibit a sympathetic leader that not only offers consistent and accurate feedback but also does so through effective communication. The leader's close connection to their team members, both on an emotional and practical level, cultivates a work atmosphere that promotes a sense of worth and comprehension among all individuals.

In her online course on vital soft skills for professional success, Raquel Roca emphasizes the importance of soft skills, irrespective of an individual's profession or employment position. The author contends that enhancing one's soft skills is the most significant action one can undertake to enhance their professional image. The possession of these soft talents is of utmost importance for a leader who demonstrates empathy, as they enable teams to effectively achieve their goals and adhere to established timelines. By enhancing their problem-solving and decision-making capabilities, individuals establish a foundation for achieving favorable outcomes. Hence, the acquisition of leadership training holds immense value for individuals who aspire to exemplify the characteristics of a genuinely sympathetic leader.

Transformational leadership: is a crucial aspect of effective leadership, when empathetic leaders strive to enhance their talents in order to effectively guide and inspire others. Could you perhaps provide further context or specify what "this" refers to? Encourage and foster inspiration among individuals while actively embracing change and actively pursuing innovative approaches in order to cultivate enjoyment.

Organization, planning, and self-management tools: are crucial for attaining the objectives of projects in which empathic leaders and their teams are involved.

The Significance of Storytelling: The Importance of Content and Delivery in Empathetic Leadership. Due to this rationale, the art of storytelling emerges as an exceedingly desirable skill that may be further cultivated through leadership courses tailored for corporate entities.

8: Promote Respect among team members

The encouragement of respect among those in the team at work is another area where an empathic leader and a boss vary. To actually have a beneficial effect on individuals, it is crucial that it begin from within the organizational culture.

As a result, there may be an improvement in the working environment, allowing team members to communicate more amicably and succinctly in order to accomplish the objective as a unit.

The truth is that when individuals feel that their opinions are being heard, they can speak more clearly and feel more inspired to take part in activities like the company's digital transformation.

How can I lead with empathy and foster respect? To help you with this, consider the following advice:

Attend meetings on time. If there are frequently delays or, on the other side, there are unlikely to be delays at all, it suggests that the meeting isn't significant enough to take place.

Greeting everyone at the start of the working day or at a meeting is an essential element in developing into a compassionate boss. Teams do not consist of "robots"; instead, members need to be more sympathetic and human in order to cooperate toward shared goals.

Provide forums for discussion: Empathic leaders do not offer responsibilities with the addition of a lack of communication. On the other hand, some leaders aim to empower their team by involving them in decision-making, the creation of strategies, the distribution of tasks, or the manner in which the work process will be implemented for each specific project.

Express interest in what the other person is saying: an effective technique for getting this message across to the other person is to paraphrase. This means that as an empathic leader, you can pay attention to what a team member says in a meeting and elaborate on the issue or concept he has raised.

9: Arrange effective team meetings

The significance of upholding efficient communication has become increasingly apparent in light of the changing work environment characterized by the emergence of distant and hybrid work models. Frequent meetings are commonly observed in such setups due to the apprehension that geographically scattered teams may need more cohesiveness and alignment with their objectives in the absence of regular in-person encounters. However, the crucial factor lies not in the frequency of meetings but in their effectiveness.

A leader who possesses empathy acknowledges the significance of their team's time and carefully considers the importance of each meeting. They consistently inquire: Is this meeting indispensable? Is it possible to accomplish its intended objective by means of a basic electronic mail message? Regardless of team members' dispersed work locations, as stated by Emily Rose McRae, a notable person working with the company known as Gartner, leaders are responsible for creating policies that support the development of connections among team members. This emphasizes the idea that the importance of a link is determined more by its quality than its quantity.

A saying that highlights the worth of time as an invaluable asset must be kept in mind. Meetings that provide little value and serve to consume time can impede productivity. Effective leaders should possess a comprehensive understanding of the underlying purpose, frequency, and objectives of meetings while exercising discernment when extending invitations. In addition, it is advantageous for teams to employ tools that facilitate the organization of meetings through the identification of shared availability, thus preventing scheduling conflicts and minimizing the need for agenda adjustments.

Furthermore, an article from Forbes emphasizes a crucial aspect of successful meetings: promoting active engagement and minimizing digressive conversations. Through embodying empathic leadership, one has the potential to enhance the efficacy of meetings by encouraging the active participation of attendees, urging them to arrive well-prepared with relevant contributions pertaining to the subject at hand.

10: Master the art of writing clear and direct emails:

It is advisable to refrain from using roundabouts in email communication. This technology greatly aids the creation of information and data sharing among employees within the organization. However, mistakes can happen occasionally, which can cause interaction issues, demand more effort and time, and eventually result in a reduction in performance.

Employing an exciting subject matter that summarizes the communication's main point is essential to writing brief and to-the-point emails. Similarly, it's crucial to use a professional accent and ensure the information is thorough, concentrated, clear, and unambiguous. Each of these elements helps to create compassionate leadership abilities.

Choosing the people who should get the email is another key consideration. Should it be distributed to all members of a team or only specific individuals?

Assuming a leadership position entails significant accountability. However, prioritizing the perspectives and emotions of one's team members makes it feasible to effectively steer them toward becoming leaders in their own right. It is crucial to prioritize effective communication while also demonstrating honesty and integrity in one's actions.

"An organization where people can exist as themselves, where they have influence, where they align with the purpose of the company, is going to be an organization that allows them to thrive. Leadership makes it possible or unattainable."

How To Spot People Who Do Not Have Empathy

Because of the complexities of their causes, empathy issues can be difficult to identify with certainty. However, some behaviors are clear indicators of lack of empathy and should prompt you to consider taking action.

- Accusing others of mistakes

- Saying others are overly sensitive: We all do it occasionally, but people who do not empathize do it far more frequently and in far more situations.

- Refusing to listen to other people's points of view

- Argumentative demeanor

- Seems to have difficulty understanding where other people are coming from.

- Can't deal with emotional situations

Reactions that are unexpectedly emotional: Typically manifest as strong feelings of frustration or even anger, stemming from their lack of understanding of and impatience with other people's feelings.

Maintaining relationships is difficult.

It is certainly worth your effort to address the situation if you think someone you know lacks empathy. Depending on the source, different amounts of patience and difficulty are needed. It is simpler to cope with unempathetic coworkers or casual social acquaintances than it is to deal with intimate friends or family members. But some instruments can handle any circumstance.

First, remember that the actions aren't necessarily driven by malice. It might be the outcome of severe trauma or personal pain, and overcoming it will take time and effort on many different levels. Adjusting emotional pathways takes weeks, if not months, instead of more surface-level behavior change.

Encouraging open dialogue

Empathy gaps may result from a confluence of unconsciously held beliefs and social forces. Many people internalize hurt because they worry about coming out as overly sensitive. They might use the excuse that it's just the way they are to minimize someone else's sarcasm: "That's the way he is." The idea is to confront it squarely. When someone seems distant or disinterested, it's critical to communicate your feelings. Finding solutions and affirming feelings are the goals here rather than assigning blame.

Being patient is crucial.

Empathy, or lack thereof, has a long history. Give change time even after addressing the problem. Depending on your connection, you could display different levels of patience. Reminders with coworkers may be necessary, but cooperation with loved ones is necessary.

Keep Your Boundaries.

Establishing clear limits is essential for open communication and patience. People who have trouble empathizing might not be aware of these boundaries unless they are made explicit. They might unintentionally go too far. Setting and upholding your boundaries is therefore crucial.

Be willing to walk away

Sometimes, relationships don't get better. No matter how desperately you try, knowing when to let go is essential in these circumstances.

Interacting with people who really lack empathetic thinking especially those who have serious psychological issues, can be draining. Realizing a relationship is poisonous is not an indicator of failure. It's not a sign of failure to realize a relationship is toxic.

The challenge of lacking empathy

Being out of rhythm with others is uncomfortable for everyone. We all yearn for connection and understanding. This relies heavily on empathy. Establishing relationships becomes a herculean endeavor when it is absent. And without it, life is unquestionably harder. In such cases, professional advice might be extremely helpful. Even if achieving full empathy may be impossible, learning its nuances can have a huge impact.

Why do Some leaders neglect empathy?

According to research, hubris syndrome can result from a brain rewiring process brought on by power. Leaders frequently struggle with extreme pressure, which forces them to give priority to measurable accomplishments above empathic acts. The importance of empathy could seem elusive given the pressure to perform. Furthermore, it is impossible to fake true empathy. Furthermore, leaders who fake it are exposed, and it frequently backfires. For many people, delving deeply into emotional spheres can be disconcerting. Leaders may be hesitant to deal with strong emotions out of concern that they may become overwhelmed. Finally, historically, leaders have given systems more importance than personal wants. They could wonder, "Why take a soft stance right now?"

Taking Care of the Empathy Gap

Do these arguments make sense? The attitude of the leadership frequently establishes the tone of the organization. Consider the leadership clues if your organization lacks empathy. There is a strong commercial case for empathy. The path can be paved through the introduction of executive coaching, particularly at the leadership level. The objective is sincere effort, not perfection.

CONCLUSION

Empathy serves as a fundamental pillar of influential leadership. The revitalization of the workplace is facilitated by the cultivation of teamwork, positivism, and enhanced comprehension. Therefore, in order to cultivate a peaceful work environment and foster authentic team cohesion, it is imperative to have leaders who actively embrace and demonstrate empathy. I truly hope that readers of this book will recognize empathy's critical role in all facets of military leadership. Our objective is a reminder of how crucial it is to comprehend those who have sacrificed everything to serve. I'm adamant that when they pledge to serve with selflessness, people need fair, kind, reliable, and, most importantly, empathic leaders. Being military leaders does not excuse us from upholding the fundamental tenets of our line of work to provide a sympathetic ear or emotional support to someone who shares our commitment to our country. The phrase "Mission first, People always" perfectly encapsulates empathy. Empathy is innovative, courageous, and free of prejudice. Start acting now, leaders and service members. All service members can gain from incorporating empathy into their professional settings and terminology, even though this book largely discusses the role of leadership in the military, this book is about the employment of empathy at all levels of the military for *Empathy has no Rank*.

ABOUT THE AUTHOR

Dr. Raheem Lay, a profound believer in the transformative power of empathy, is not just an advocate but an embodiment of emotional intelligence. With a combined 22 years in therapy-related education, including a master's, doctorate in social work, and a certification in Empathy and Emotional Intelligence Coaching, he has dedicated his life to bettering human connection. He currently extends his expertise as a Mental Health Provider for the U.S. Air Force. In 2022, Dr. Lay founded courses on empathy for various professionals, highlighting his commitment to education. He resides in San Antonio, enjoying family moments and occasional social media engagements.

www.ingramcontent.com/pod-product-compliance
Lightning Source LLC
Chambersburg PA
CBHW020445220526
45464CB00002B/872